130/254819
23.11.79

£21.20

D1338417

Recent Results in Cancer Research 66

Fortschritte der Krebsforschung
Progrès dans les recherches sur le cancer

Edited by

V. G. Allfrey, New York · M. Allgöwer, Basel
I. Berenblum, Rehovoth · F. Bergel, Jersey
J. Bernard, Paris · W. Bernhard, Villejuif
N. N. Blokhin, Moskva · H. E. Bock, Tübingen
W. Braun, New Brunswick · P. Bucalossi, Milano
A. V. Chaklin, Moskva · M. Chorazy, Gliwice
G. J. Cunningham, Richmond · G. Della Porta, Milano
P. Denoix, Villejuif · R. Dulbecco, La Jolla
H. Eagle, New York · R. Eker, Oslo
R. A. Good, New York · P. Grabar, Paris
R. J. C. Harris, Salisbury · E. Hecker, Heidelberg
R. Herbeuval, Vandoeuvre · J. Higginson, Lyon
W. C. Hueper, Fort Myers · H. Isliker, Lausanne
J. Kieler, Kobenhavn · W. H. Kirsten, Chicago
G. Klein, Stockholm · H. Koprowski, Philadelphia
L. G. Koss, New York · G. Martz, Zürich
G. Mathé, Villejuif · O. Mühlbock, Amsterdam
W. Nakahara, Tokyo · L. J. Old, New York
V. R. Potter, Madison · A. B. Sabin, Charleston, S.C.
L. Sachs, Rehovoth · E. A. Saxén, Helsinki
C. G. Schmidt, Essen · S. Spiegelman, New York
W. Szybalski, Madison · H. Tagnon, Bruxelles
R. M. Taylor, Toronto · A. Tissières, Genève
E. Uehlinger, Zürich · R. W. Wissler, Chicago

Editor in Chief: P. Rentchnick, Genève

Carcinogenic Hormones

Edited by C. H. Lingeman

With 156 Figures and 24 Tables

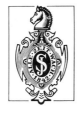

Springer-Verlag
Berlin Heidelberg New York 1979

Carolyn H. Lingeman, M.D.

Division of Cancer Cause and Prevention
National Cancer Institute
Bethesda, MD 20014 and
Department of Environmental and
Drug Induced Pathology
Armed Forces Institute of Pathology
Washington, DC 20306/USA

Sponsored by the Swiss League against Cancer

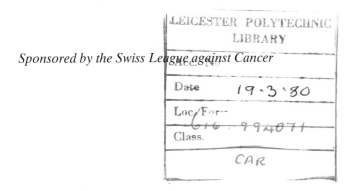

ISBN 3-540-08995-0 Springer-Verlag Berlin Heidelberg New York
ISBN 0-387-08995-0 Springer-Verlag New York Heidelberg Berlin

Library of Congress Cataloging in Publication Data. Main entry under title: Carcino-
genic hormones. (Recent results in cancer research; 66)
Proceedings of a symposium sponsored by the Swiss League Against Cancer. 1. Steroid
hormones—Toxicology—Congresses. 2. Carcinogens—Congresses. I. Lingeman, Carolyn H.
II. Schweizerische Nationalliga für Krebsbekämpfung und Krebsforschung. III. Series.
[DNLM: 1. Hormones—Adverse effects—Congresses. 2. Estrogens—effects—Congresses. 3. Neoplasms—Etiology—Congresses. 4. Carcinogens—Congresses. W1
RE106P v. 66/QZ202.3 C265 1976] RC261.R35 no. 66 [RC268.7.S7]
616.9'94'008s [616.9'94'071] 78-12072

© Springer-Verlag Berlin · Heidelberg 1979

Printed in Germany

The use of registered names, trademarks, etc. in the publication does not imply,
even in the absence of a specific statement, that such names are exempt from the
relevant protective laws and regulations and therefore free for general use.

Typesetting, printing, and binding: Carl Ritter & Co./Wiesbaden

2125/3140—5 4 3 2 1 0

Foreword

Either deficient or excessive hormone production has been observed with respect to some rather bizarre clinical manifestations. Starting with the synthesis or isolation of pure hormones in the early 30s, estrogens (the female sex hormones) and androgens (the male sex hormones) have become readily available for clinical and other uses and their physiologic activity has been intensively studied. The relationship between hormones and cancer was perhaps one of the earliest research areas in cancer. In the early work of the 20s it was clearly shown in experimental animals that under certain conditions both endogenous and exogenous hormones could induce certain cancers and tumors.

More recently, attention has been focused on the use of androgenic anabolic steroids by athletes as body builders and the widescale multiple use of estrogens in terms of carcinogenic hazard. Most striking in recent years are the potential adverse effects of estrogens relevant to sterility, gall bladder disease, and neoplasia. The pervasive environmental hazard contributed by estrogens may arise from variant sources. Such sources may be: (a) endogenous hormones, (b) estrogenic compounds occurring naturally in foods or as fungal contaminants in food stuffs, (c) estrogens added to livestock feed, (d) estrogenic additives to cosmetics, (e) oral contraceptives, and (f) estrogens used clinically for threatened abortions, lactation suppression, menstrual anomalies, and therapeutic treatment of certain forms of cancer.

The revelation of the potential carcinogenic risk from estrogens used as feed supplements and the most recent discovery of the latent effects of some of the above delineated medical uses have been cause for much concern. Because of this extensive concern, a two-day symposium was conducted under the auspices of the Interagency Collaborative Group on Environmental Carcinogenesis, an interagency group sponsored by the National Cancer Institute. It was deemed appropriate that the proceedings of this symposium be made available to a larger audience than those participating, hence the publication of this monograph.

H. F. Kraybill, Ph.D.
Chairman, Interagency Collaborative
    Group on Environmental Carcinogenesis
National Cancer Institute
Bethesda, MD 20014 / USA

Acknowledgments

Dr. NELSON S. IREY, Chairman, Department of Environmental and Drug Induced Pathology, Armed Forces Institute of Pathology, Washington, D. C., and Dr. WILLIAM D'AGUANNO, Bureau of Drugs, Food and Drug Administration, Washington, D. C. assisted in planning the programs that resulted in the preparation of this monograph. Dr. IREY reviewed some of the manuscripts.

Contents

List of Contributors

H. W. Casey, D.V.M., Ph.D., Chairman, Department of Veterinary Pathology, Armed Forces Institute of Pathology, Washington, DC 20306/USA

T. B. Dunn, M.D., Consultant, Registry of Experimental Cancers, National Cancer Institute, National Institutes of Health, Bethesda, MD 20014/USA

R. C. Giles, D.V.M., Diagnostic Laboratory, Kentucky Department of Agriculture, North Drive, Hopkinsville, KY 42240/USA

G. D. Hilliard, M.D., Department of Gynecologic and Breast Pathology, Armed Forces Institute of Pathology, Washington, DC 20306/USA

K. G. Ishak, M.D., Ph.D., Chairman, Department of Hepatic Pathology, Armed Forces Institute of Pathology, Washington, DC 20306/USA

R. J. Kurman, M.D., Georgetown University, School of Medicine, Departments of Pathology and Obstetrics and Gynecology, 3800 Reservoir Road, Washington, DC 20007/USA

R. P. Kwapien, D.V.M., Ph.D., Department of Pathology and Parisitology, School of Veterinary Medicine, Auburn University, Auburn, AL 36830/USA

C. H. Lingeman, M.D., Division of Cancer Cause and Prevention, National Cancer Institute, Bethesda, MD 20014 and Department of Environmental and Drug Induced Pathology, Armed Forces Institute of Pathology, Washington, DC 20306/USA

H. J. Norris, M.D., Chairman, Department of Gynecologic and Breast Pathology, Armed Forces Institute of Pathology, Washington, DC 20306/USA

Hormones and Hormonomimetic Compounds in the Etiology of Cancer

Carolyn H. Lingeman[1]

Hormones, particularly those produced by the gonads, and their synthetic analogs have been the subject of controversy concerning their roles in the process of carcinogenesis. Experimental evidence, dating from 1916 [118] (Table 1), that estrogens can be potent carcinogens was overlooked or lightly dismissed by many because of a prevalent belief that the body should be able to metabolize these physiologic compounds without toxic effects. The relevance of animal experiments to the human cancer problem was also questioned. During the past four decades, a variety of naturally occurring and synthetic estrogens, progestins, and androgens have been manufactured and prescribed in ever-increasing amounts for replacement, treatment of cancer, prevention of abortion, suppression of lactation, contraception, and other purposes without adequate attention to their carcinogenic potential.

Cancer of the vagina and cervix of women exposed to diethylstilbestrol (DES) in utero might have been anticipated if more attention had been given to reports of neoplasms in the vagina and cervix of mice given DES and other estrogens by SUNTZEFF et al. in 1938 [197] and by GARDNER and ALLEN in 1939 [64]. The same issue of the journal with the latter report [64] also contained one of the earliest reports describing DES treatment of a surgically castrated 42-year-old woman [122].

Likewise, proliferative lesions in livers of rats and mice receiving some component steroids of oral contraceptives noted in the 1960s [29] should have received more attention. These observations turned out to be prophetic when hepatocellular neoplasms occurred in women using oral contraceptives and in patients receiving androgens for anemia and other conditions.

If all this evidence is not enough to convince even the most ardent skeptics that hormones and hormonomimetic compounds can be potent carcinogens, reports linking cancer of the endometrium with long-term use of estrogens for replacement and contraception and cancer of the breast with replacement estrogens are additional ominous warnings. Agencies charged with control of the manufacture of these products and physicians who prescribe them are in particularly difficult situations for there is great public demand for "pills" to solve many problems from overpopulation to protection from the supposed ravages of age. These demands are encouraged by ingenious members of the pharmaceutical industry who anticipate the needs, suggest additional ones, and design methods to manufacture new compounds.

This monograph deals mainly with carcinogenic effects of gonadal hormones and hormonomimetic compounds because they have been well studied and their effects on target organs are

1 I am indebted to Drs. HAROLD L. STEWART, HERMAN F. KRAYBILL, and ERWIN P. VOLLMER for their helpful comments and suggestions.

Table 1. Significant historical events in hormonal carcinogenesis

1713	Ramazzini noted an apparent high frequency of breast cancer in nuns [62].
1842	Rigoni-Stern confirmed the high frequency of breast cancer in nuns and other unmarried women [62].
1896	Beatson reported clinical improvement of human breast cancer following surgical castration [13].
1916	Mouse mammary gland neoplasms prevented by early castration [118].
1929	Estrone extracted from urine of pregnant women [41].
1932	Lacassagne induced carcinoma of the mammary gland in male mice by injecting folliculin [117].
1938	Dodds et al. reported estrogenic activity of a nonsteroid compound, diethylstilbestrol (DES) [40].
1938—1939	Reports of carcinogenicity of several estrogens, including DES, in vagina and cervix of mice [64, 197].
1939	DES prescribed for estrogen replacement in a surgically castrated women [122].
1941	Commercial production of DES reported [97].
1946	DES advocated as treatment for so-called high-risk pregnancies [190].
1947	DES implants permitted in poultry for "caponization" in the United States [108].
1948	U.S. Food and Drug Administration (FDA) regulation published in the *Federal Register* stating that no residues of DES should remain in edible tissues [108].
1954	DES at levels of 10 mg/head/day permitted to be fed to beef cattle in the United States [108].
1955	DES implants in ears of beef cattle permitted in the United States [108].
1958	Enactment of U.S. law ("Delaney clause") prohibiting use of materials with carcinogenic activity as food additives [108].
1959	DES implants in poultry prohibited in the United States because of residues in livers [108].
1962	"Delaney clause" amended permitting use of potential carcinogens in food animals providing no residues are detectable in meat from such animals [108].
1971	Report of vaginal adenocarcinoma in women exposed to DES in utero [87].
1971	Report of hepatocellular carcinoma in a patient receiving anabolic steroids [198].
1972	Hepatocellular neoplasms reported in rats given steroid components of oral contraceptives [29].
1973	Hepatocellular neoplasms reported in women using oral contraceptives [12].
1973—1974	U.S. FDA banned use of DES in food animals; the ban was later overturned by U.S. Court of Appeals on the grounds that manufactures of DES were denied a hearing [108].
1975	U.S. Senate Committee hearings resulted in a request for ban on use of DES in food animals and medical uses (with a few exceptions) [108].
1975	Report of increased risk of adenocarcinoma of the endometrium in women using exogenous estrogens [189, 212], including the sequential type of oral contraceptive [131].
1976	Notice by FDA of proposal to withdraw New Animal Drug Applications for DES published in the U.S. *Federal Register* [108].

readily measurable. Hormones secreted by other organs may be equally or more significant in carcinogenesis, but knowledge of their activity and possible roles in the etiology of cancer is in a more primitive state at the present time. Furthermore, because this monograph deals only with the *etiologic* aspects of hormones, many interesting facts about their activities have been omitted because a relation to the induction of cancer is not evident. Tables 2 and 3 indicate hormones that have been implicated as carcinogens in man or animals.

Chemistry, Biology and Pharamcology

Published material relating to the chemistry and biologic activity of hormones is abundant, but it is difficult to determine which is relevant to the *etiology* of cancer. Several reviews have summarized many of the significant facts on this subject, most notably the monograph produced by the International Agency for Research on Cancer (IARC) [97] and an article by HERTZ [89]. Formulas for some compounds that may be significant in carcinogenesis are given in Figures 1—8. Most of the formulas and common or trivial names are those listed in the 9th edition of *The Merck Index* [144]. Some commercial hormone products are mixtures of hormones in variable proportions. For example, most oral contraceptives are composed of a synthetic steroidal estrogen combined with a synthetic progestin (Table 4). The conjugated equine steroidal product Premarin is composed of sulfates of several estrogens, including some that appear to be formed only by equine species [144]. Such products in tablet form contain coloring agents and other materials that may also contribute to their carcinogenicity.

In vivo, the main starting material in the biosynthesis of steroid hormones is *cholesterol,* which is formed from acetate ions by enzymatic synthesis [97, 200]. The primary synthetic reactions involve partial or complete degradation of the side chain attached to carbon atom 17 of the cholesterol molecule and the incorporation of oxygen atoms. More than 90% of plasma steroids are bound to proteins such as serum albumin, α- and β-glycoproteins, various globulins, and other proteins [136]. Testosterone and estradiol-17β are transported by the same steroid-binding β-globulin. The synthesis of this globulin is regulated by thyroid hormones [135]. Inactivation of steroids in the liver mainly involves the uptake of hydrogen to saturate double bonds and reduction of keto to hydroxyl groups. Water soluble conjugates are formed with sulfates and glucuronides for excretion in urine or bile.

Commercial production of steroid hormones also begins with cholesterol or other suitable precursor compounds derived from wool fat, cattle bile, or plant steroids such as *diosgenin* (Fig. 1). These steroids are transformed by chemical or biologic reactions that add or subtract ions or radicals to obtain the desired qualities. Bacterial or fungal enzymes can perform some of the chemical reactions such as hydroxylation and cleavage of side chains [205]. The manufacture of hormone products often requires the development of sophisticated chemical reactions to achieve the desired qualities. For example, the so-called anabolic steroids are androgens in which the anabolic effects are retained but the masculinizing properties are eliminated or minimized. Selection of a compound for manufacture may also involve such nonscientific considerations as patent rights and availability of raw materials.

Table 2. Hormone preparations reported to induce neoplasms

Hormone	Human	Animals		
		Mice	Rats	Other
Estrogens:				
Conjugated equine	Endometrium [212] Breast [93]		MG [97] Pit. [97] UB [97]	Kidney in hamsters [97] Ovary in dogs [97, 164] Uterus in squirrel monkeys [97]
Diethyl-stilbestrol (DES)	Vagina, cervix [87]a,b Ovary [94] Endometrium [36, 92]	MG [97] Vagina-cervix [97, 197] Testes [187] Lymphoid tissue [97]		
Estrone		MG [97]	MG [97] Adrenal [97] Pit. [97] UB [97]	Kidney in hamsters [97]
Estradiol-17β		MG [97] Uterus [97] Vagina [97] Testes [97] Pit. [97] Lymphoid tissue [97]	MG [97] Pit. [97]	Kidney in hamsters [97]
Estriol		MG [174]	Adrenal cortex [158, 159]	
Mestranol	Liverc [12, 172]	MG [97] Pit. [97] Vagina-cervixb [97]	MG [97] Liverb [29]	
Ethynylestradiol	Liverc [12, 172] Endometriumd [131, 188]	MG [97] Pit. [97] Uterus [97]	Liverb [97]	

Metabolism of Steroids

Despite their diverse chemical structures and biologic activity, most steroids, whether endogenous or synthetic, undergo similar conjugation and excretion. Conjugated and unconjugated steroids and their metabolites are excreted in urine and feces, the proportions

Progestins:			
Progesterone	MGe [97] Ovary [97] Uterus [97]		MG in dogsf [97]
Chlormadinone acetate	MGe [97] Pit.e [97]		MG in dogsf [97]
Medroxy-progesterone acetate			
Norethisterone	Liver [97] Ovary [97] Pit. [97]	Liver [97]	
Norethynodrel	Pit. [97] MG [97]	Pit. [97] MG [97] Liver [97]	
Androgens:			
Methyl-testosterone	Liver [52, 198]		
Testosterone	Uterus [97]		
Oxymetholone	Liver [52, 198]		

a Also hexestrol and dienestrol.
b See KURMAN, this monograph.
c Combined with a progestin.
d Used in a sequential type of oral contraceptive.
e Combined with an estrogen.
f See CASEY et al. this monograph.
Abbreviations: MG = mammary gland; Pit. = pituitary gland; UB = urinary bladder.

depending on the species of animal and the characteristics of the compound. Conjugation of steroids to sulfates and glucuronates occurs primarily in the liver and a large proportion of conjugated steroids is secreted in the bile. Some fecal steroids are reabsorbed in the intestine and thus reenter the metabolic pool of interacting compounds. In the liver, detoxification of both endogenous and exogenous hormones is accomplished by enzymes of the same types

Table 3. Commercial hormone preparations reported to be human carcinogens

Hormone	Marketed	Uses	Exposure	Location of neoplasm	Histologic type of neoplasm
Estrogens:					
Conjugated equine steroids	1930s	Replacement	Women, middle age or older	Uterine endometrium	Adenocarcinoma [212]
				Breast	Carcinoma [93]
DES	1930s	Replacement	Young women with gonadal dysgenesis	Endometrium	Adenocarcinoma [36]
			Mainly older women		
		Threatened abortion[a]	Early fetal life	Ovary	Carcinoma [94]
				Vagina, cervix	Clear-cell adenocarcinoma [87]
		Treatment for breast cancer	Mostly older women	Endometrium	Adenocarcinoma [92]
Mestranol, ethynyl-estradiol	1960s	Contraception	Mainly young women	Liver	Hepatocellular adenoma, carcinoma [12, 172][b]
				Endometrium	Adenocarcinoma [131, 188][c]
Androgens:					
Methyltestosterone	1940s	Replacement	Males, all ages	Liver	Hepatocellular neoplasms [52, 198][d]
		Anemia	Mainly children, male and female	Liver	Hepatocellular neoplasms [52, 198][d]
Anabolic steroids (oxymetholone and others)	1960s	Anemia	Mainly children, male and female	Liver	Hepatocellular neoplasms [52, 198][d]

[a] Also hexestrol and dienestrol (see KURMAN, this monograph).
[b] In most reported cases the estrogen was combined with a synthetic progestin.
[c] Most occurred in users of the sequential type of oral contraception (see HILLIARD and NORRIS, this monograph).
[d] The precise nature of these neoplasms remains to be determined [198]. Some were reversible after cessation of use of the drug (see ISHAK, this monograph).

that metabolize and detoxify a variety of chemical compounds including many drugs [33], a topic that is discussed more fully in another paragraph. These drug-metabolizing enzymes also activate carcinogens. Hormones can induce or compete for hydroxylating enzymes and interact with other compounds in ways that are difficult to predict. Hormones also compete

Table 4. Classification of some hormonally active compounds[a]

Classification	Steroid		Nonsteroid	
	Naturally occurring	Synthetic	Naturally occurring	Synthetic
Estrogenic	Estriol[b] Estrone[b] Estradiol[b] Equilin[c] Equilenin[c]	Mestranol Ethynylestradiol	Phytoestrogens: Coumestrol Genistein Zearalenone	Diethylstilbestrol (DES) Hexestrol Dienestrol Chlorotrianisene
Progestational	Progesterone[b]	17-hydroxyprogesterones: Medroxyprogesterone acetate Chlormadinone acetate Megestrol acetate 19-nortestosterone derivatives: Dimethisterone Ethynerone Ethynodiol diacetate Norethindrone (Norethisterone) Norethynodrel Norgestrel		
Androgenic (anabolic)	Testosterone[b] 5α-dihydrotestosterone (DHT)	Oxymetholone Norethandrolone 17-methyltestosterone		
Other: Anti-androgen		Cyproterone		

[a] Trivial names listed first in the 9th edition of *The Merck Index* [144]. Formulas are given in Figures 1–8.
[b] Can be synthesized from other steroids.
[c] Believed to occur only in equine species.

with other chemical compounds for receptor sites in cells. In aging rats, the capacity to induce some drug-metabolizing enzymes decreases [2]. Decreased capacity for critical enzyme adaptations required for life processes may have a bearing on the higher frequencies of many diseases occurring in advanced ages.

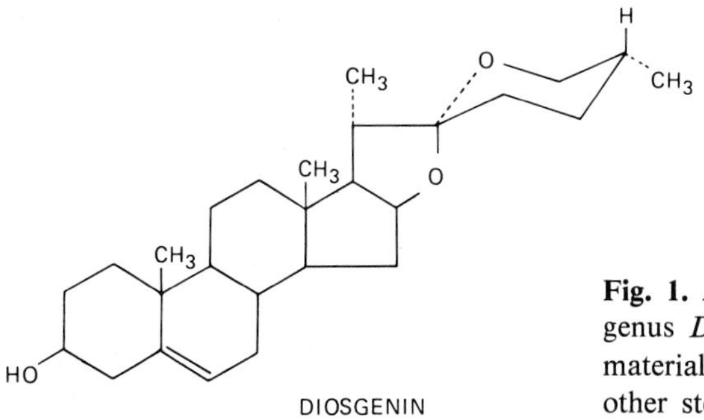

CH₃

DIOSGENIN

Fig. 1. An aglycone extracted from plants of the genus *Dioscorea* used commercially as a raw material in the synthesis of progesterones and other steroids

Estrogens

Controlled primarily by pituitary gonadotropins, the three main endogenous estrogens, *estrone, estradiol,* and *estriol* (Fig. 2), are formed in the ovary, placenta, testes, and adrenal glands, mainly from cholesterol. They are also formed in other tissues such as body fat and brain by conversion of nonestrogenic steroids such as *testosterone* and *androstenedione*. Circulating estrogens, primarily bound to protein, are processed in the liver by several mechanisms including hydroxylation and conjugation with glucuronic and sulfuric acids for excretion in urine or bile. Both exogenous and endogenous estrogens are stored in body fat [71]. Estrogens are antagonistic to testosterone, but to progesterone they can be synergistic or antagonistic. Estrogenic activity is assessed by measuring the increase in uterine weight of rodents compared to a standard estrogen or by noting the degree of cornification of cells of vaginal epithelium, both biologic methods that are difficult to quantitate. Newer techniques such as radioimmunoassay permit more accurate quantitation of these compounds.

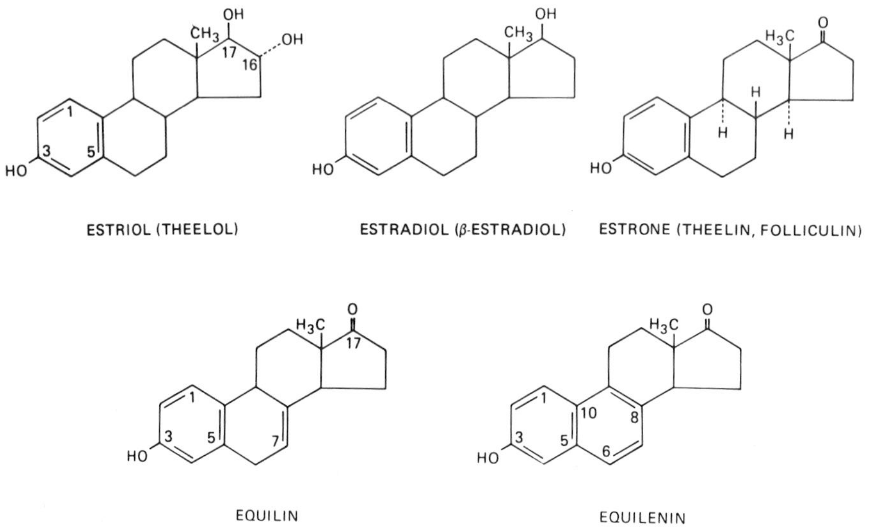

ESTRIOL (THEELOL)   ESTRADIOL (β-ESTRADIOL)   ESTRONE (THEELIN, FOLLICULIN)

EQUILIN   EQUILENIN

Fig. 2. Naturally occurring steroidal estrogens

While estrogens are mainly concerned with reproduction and are believed to be produced by all vertebrates, the presence of estrogen receptors in organs other than those of the female genital system and mammary glands indicates that they participate in a broader spectrum of activities than those directly concerned with conceiving and nourishing offspring. Estrogens affect bone (ossification of epiphyses and maintenance of bone integrity), plasma lipids and coagulation factors, the biliary system, blood vessels, lymphoid organs, and many other tissues.

Synthetic estrogens are steroids and nonsteroidal compounds with biologic action that mimics that of endogenous estrogens. They may be derived from other steroids or synthesized by other reactions. In 1938, DODDS et al. [40] reported that a nonsteroidal compound, diethylstilbestrol (DES) (Fig. 3), demonstrated biologic activity qualitatively similar to that of estrogens extracted from the ovary. Unlike estrogens extracted from equine urine available at the time and requiring injection or implantation, DES was effective when given orally. It was more potent than ovarian estrogens, the dosage could be regulated more accurately, and it could be manufactured more cheaply. It was subsequently found to be bound by the same cell receptor proteins as estradiol. The biologic activity of DES, a stilbene, is believed to depend on the presence of free hydroxyl groups; conjugation of these groups with glucuronic acid results in a marked decrease in uterotropic activity [139]. The biologic activity of DES also depends on the position of the methyl groups in the molecule relative to the phenolic hydroxyls, the length of the alkyl groups, and the isomeric structure (*trans*-DES is more active than the *cis* form) [139]. There are species differences in the *rate* of DES metabolism, but the feces is the major route of DES excretion in most species that have been studied. As with endogenous steroids, a large proportion of DES is conjugated in the liver and enters the feces via the bile. There is also some enterohepatic recirculation. Small amounts of DES are excreted in the urine.

Ethynylestradiol (Fig. 4), a synthetic steroidal estrogen, first synthesized in 1938, and its 3-methyl ether derivative *mestranol* are used primarily in oral contraceptives, but have also been used for many years for some of the same purposes as DES and other estrogens. They

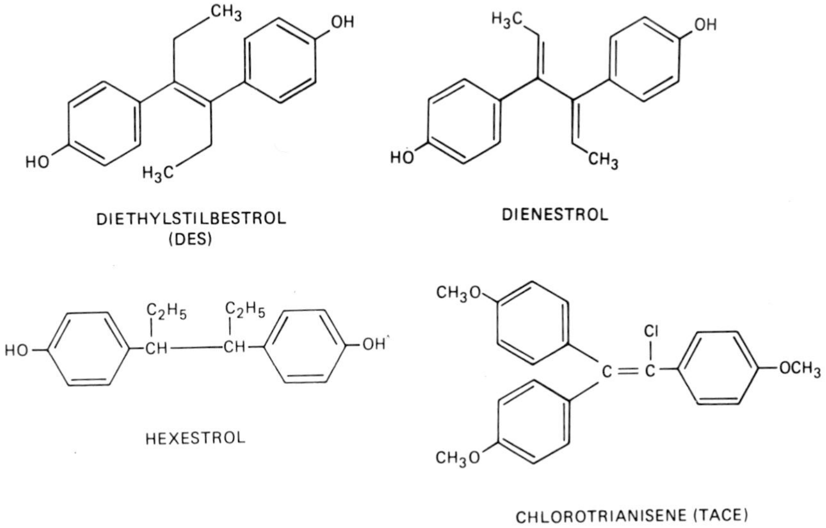

Fig. 3. Synthetic nonsteroidal compounds with estrogenic activity

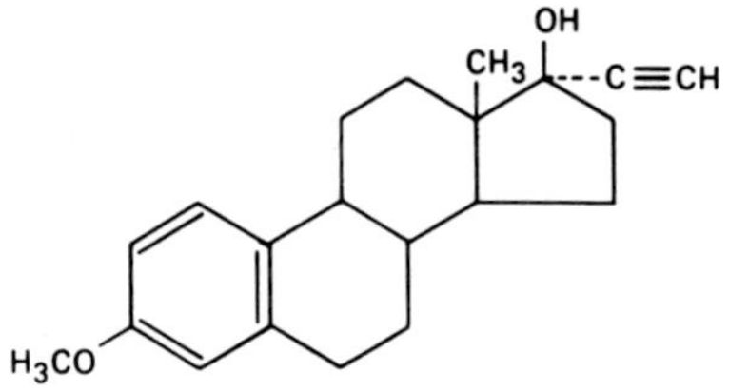

Fig. 4. Synthetic steroidal estrogens

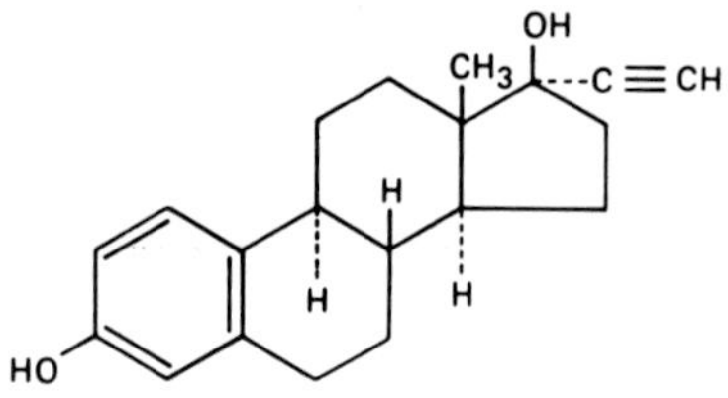

are metabolized in general by the same mechanisms as endogenous estrogens [97] although there is considerable species variation in patterns of metabolism and excretion [60]. The species variations should be considered when toxicity and carcinogenicity testing of these products is planned.

Conjugated Equine Estrogens

Premarin (Ayerst), the most widely used estrogen replacement product in the United States, is a mixture of the sodium salts of water-soluble estrogen sulfates blended to "represent the average composition of material derived from the urine of pregnant mares" [169]. It contains mostly estrone, equilin (Fig. 2), and 17α-dihydroequilin, with smaller amounts of 17α-estradiol, equilenin, and 17α-dihydroequilenin as salts of their sulfate esters [169]. Effects of equine estrogens in nonequine species have not been fully assessed. *Equilin* compounds were among the estrogens reported by GARDNER and ALLEN [64] to be carcinogenic in mice.

The development and manufacture of commercial estrogen products was a response to the legitimate expression of need by the medical profession which attempted to solve some of the most troublesome medical problems such as the tragedy of repeated abortions in childless women, the relief of frequently debilitating menopausal symptoms, possible prevention of the painful osteoporosis that afflicts thousands of elderly people, mostly women, contraception, and the treatment of cancer. The introduction of commercial estrogens was greeted enthusiastically and often uncritically by doctors and patients who, despite the lack of evidence of safety particularly during long-term use or despite questions about their effectiveness for some purposes, comsumed ever-increasing amounts of these potent compounds. Their use for contraception is particularly attractive because in addition to their effectiveness and their convenience, the menstrual cycle can be regulated. Furthermore these products prevent dysmenorrhea and often improve acne.

Whether or not exogenous estrogens can prevent osteoporosis is still controversial, but estrogens are known to affect the metabolism of calcium. Both endogenous and exogenous estrogens predispose to cholelithiasis [96]. Conjugated and synthetic estrogens increase the coagulability of the blood [195] (see HILLIARD and NORRIS, this monograph). The increased risk of myocardial infarction in women using oral contraceptives appears to contradict the widely held view that the lower frequency of myocardial infarction in women is a result of "protection" of the blood vessels by endogenous estrogens. The increased frequency of arteriosclerosis in women castrated at young ages and women past menopause has been explained by the decreased levels of circulating estrogens. Several years ago these observations led to attempts to prevent myocardial infarction in men by administration of estrogens or by castration, modes of therapy that fortunately never came into wide use. In fact, studies conducted by the U.S. Veterans Administration showed an *increased* number of deaths from cardiovascular disease in men who received DES for treatment of cancer of the prostate [204]. The possible relation between sex hormones and cardiovascular diseases is complex and will require additional studies to resolve the questions.

The effects of *cosmetic products* containing estrogens and other hormones have not been adequately evaluated. As early as 1934, systemic effects were noted when estrogens were applied to the skin of animals [147]. Testosterone and testosterone propionate applied to the skin of male rats and guinea pigs were absorbed in amounts sufficient to maintain the accessory reproductive organs of castrates or to cause their precocious development in young animals. The cosmetic industry was quick to recognize the potential for the manufacture of creams and lotions containing hormones for use by individuals afflicted with acne, balding, wrinkling, and other disorders of the skin. Yet despite the lack of scientific evidence that skin creams containing hormones actually improved any of these conditions, such products have been extremely popular in the United States. Systemic effects of face creams containing estrogens applied to the skin of animals include cornification of vaginal epithelium and increase of uterine weights in castrated female rats, a decrease in weight of testes and seminal vesicles of young male rats, and stimulation of the mammary glands of male guinea pigs [147]. Koss [111] states that facial creams containing estrogens "may have a pronounced effect on the (epithelium of human) vaginal smears". This effect is mainly an increased maturation of epithelium and is obvious only in the postmenopause when low estrogen levels normally result in a characteristic pattern of maturation. Therefore the report of EIDELSBERG [48] that vaginal epithelial maturation did not correlate with the use of these products is meaningless because the 14 women in the study were ages 18—56 years, ages at which estrogenic effects of exogenous estrogens would be masked in most women by high levels of circulating endogenous estrogens. Systematic studies of hormone-containing cosmetic products in older women are needed to resolve this point. Most estrogen-containing creams on the market are said to contain from 7,500—10,000 IU of "estrogenic substances"/oz vehicle [79]. It is not known how much is absorbed or what should be considered "normal usage". A panel appointed by the U.S. Food and Drug Administration (FDA) plans to review the evidence concerning the safety of these products probably in 1978 and welcomes comments about them. Estrogens absorbed from vaginal creams can also have systemic effects.

One nonmedical use of estrogens and other hormones that has the potential of exposing thousands of unsuspecting individuals to unknown levels of these potent compounds is the practice of adding DES or other compounds to fodder or implanting them in food animals for fattening or other purposes. This practice is illegal in many countries, but in the United States, despite the opposition of the FDA and other agencies concerned with the harmful effects, the practice continues as of this writing (Table 1). It is one of the inconsistencies of our times that a potent drug such as DES, ordinarily available only on prescription by a physician or a veterinarian, is available in unlimited amounts to farmers, ranchers, and other individuals who do not have the scientific background to understand the complex problems associated with their use. The U.S. FDA has proposed the withdrawal of all approval for use of DES as an animal growth promotor; hearings on this issue are in progress and are expected to be resolved in 1978.

Human and animal populations are exposed to a variety of exogenous materials with estrogen-mimetic action, including a variety of plant and microbial steroids and nonsteroids. These *phytoestrogens* will be discussed in a later section.

Despite all the evidence that estrogens can be carcinogenic, the precise mechanisms are still unknown. Do they promote carcinogenic action of other carcinogens or do they act directly on the genetic machinery of the cell? Does their activity in carcinogenesis involve the immune system? In support of the latter idea is the observation that estrogens, both synthetic and naturally occurring, can stimulate phagocytic activity of the reticuloendothelial system in mice whereas oophorectomy depresses it [194].

The similarities in the formulas of carcinogenic polycyclic hydrocarbons to those of steroid hormones has been noted by many investigators. The synergistic effects of polycyclic hydrocarbons and estrogens have been demonstrated by the fact that the latent period of skin tumors induced by application of 3,4-benzpyrene can be shortened and the incidence increased by simultaneous administration of estrone [6]. Likewise, carcinoma of the cervix and vagina in mice induced by local application of 3-methylcholanthrene occurs with greater frequency if a DES-cholesterol pellet is implanted S.C. after painting the cervix with the carcinogen [151].

Estrogens can induce estrogen-dependent neoplasms in nongenital organs in rats, including the adrenal cortex, salivary glands, and lymphoid tissues [159].

Progesterone and Other Progestins

Progesterone is secreted by the corpus luteum of the ovary, the placenta, and the adrenal glands (Fig. 5). Its major action during pregnancy is to prevent ovulation and to maintain implantation of the fertilized ovum. It is also required for the development of the mammary glands. Progesterone is moreover an intermediate product in the biosynthesis of other adrenal and testicular hormones. Similar to estrogens and testosterone, circulating plasma progesterone is bound to transport proteins and is inactivated in the liver. Bioassays depend on measurable proliferative changes in rabbit endometrium.

The progesterone-binding capacity of the uterus and vagina is stimulated by estrogens, but the mechanism is poorly understood [51]. Based on studies with hamster uterine strips, FABER et al. [51] proposed that interaction of estradiol with its own receptor causes translocation of the estrogen receptor complex to nuclear acceptor sites where it stimulates RNA synthesis. The increase in estrogen-dependent RNA results in an accelerated synthesis of the progesterone receptor.

Crystalline *progesterone* was first isolated in 1934 from corpora lutea of slaughtered animals [97]. Subsequently a number of synthetic steroids have been shown to have progestational activity (Figs. 5 and 6). Most of these are synthesized commercially from cholesterol or from phytosterols such as *stigmasterol* or *diosgenin*. Some progestins demonstrate androgenic or anti-estrogenic activity and are useful in treating carcinoma of the endometrium. Similarly to estrogens, progestins are widely prescribed in futile attempts to prevent abortion, but unfortunately have resulted in the masculinization of some female fetuses [200]. Synthetic progestins are mainly used for contraception, either alone or in combination with estrogens. Table 4 lists some synthetic progestins.

Synthetic progestins are metabolized in a manner similar to naturally occurring steroids although there are some differences in reactions of 19-nortestosterone derivatives compared to other types [60, 119]. The role of progestins in carcinogenesis is unclear, but because they are antagonistic to estrogens they apparently function to prevent or delay estrogen-promoted carcinomas of the endometrium and mammary gland.

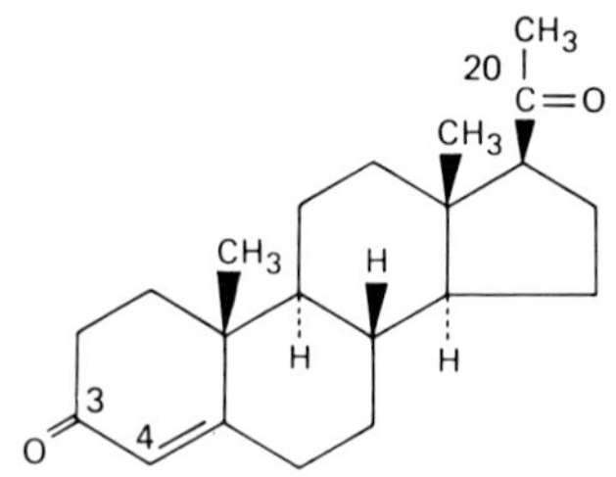

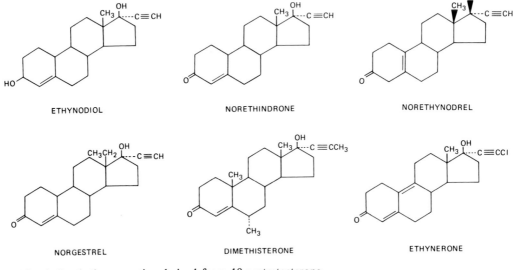

PROGESTERONE

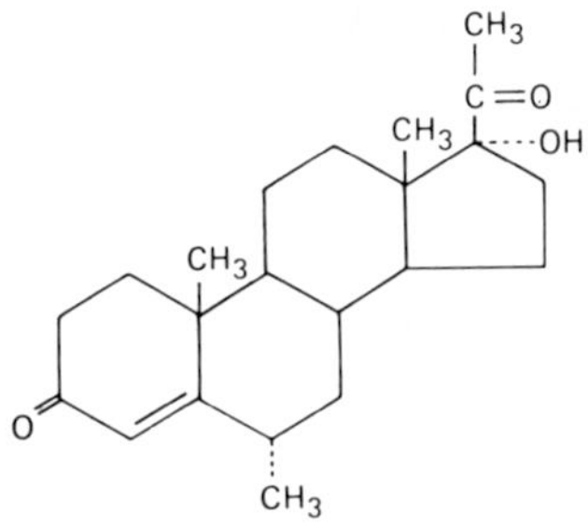

MEDROXYPROGESTERONE

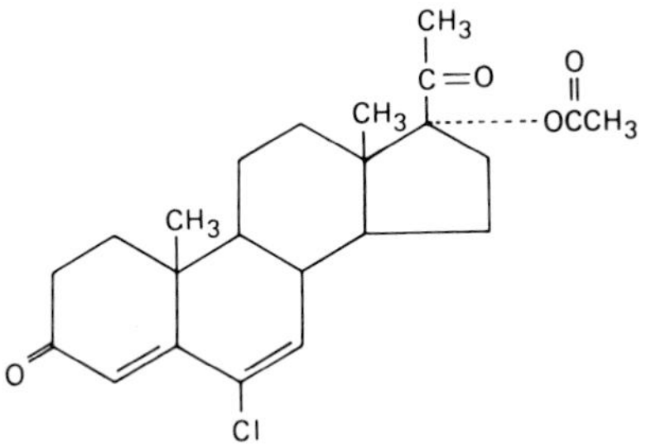

CHLORMADINONE ACETATE

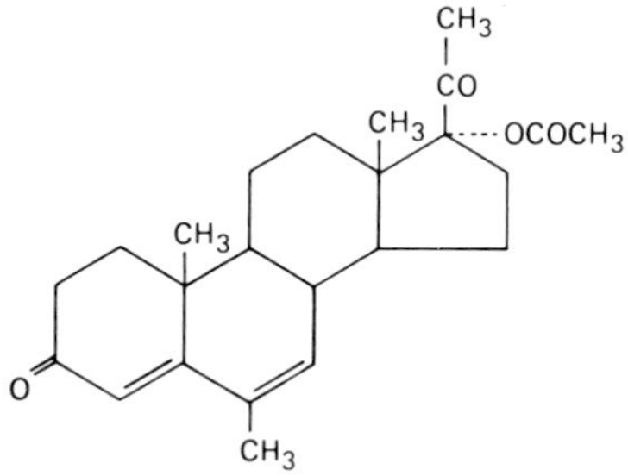

MEGESTROL ACETATE

Fig. 5. Progesterone and 17-hydroxyprogesterones

ETHYNODIOL

NORETHINDRONE

NORETHYNODREL

NORGESTREL

DIMETHISTERONE

ETHYNERONE

Fig. 6. Synthetic progestins derived from 19-nortestosterone

Androgens

Testosterone and Related Compounds

Under the control of pituitary gonadotropins, *testosterone* is formed in the testes, adrenal glands, and in small amounts in the ovaries (Fig. 7). It circulates in plasma bound to the same transport proteins that bind estrogens. Only the free fraction is biologically active. Metabolic degradation occurs primarily in the liver. The principal metabolites are 17-keto-steroids, the hydroxyl group at C-17 having been oxidized to a keto-group. One important metabolite excreted in the urine is androsterone. In both sexes, 17-keto-steroids are also formed from other steroids, mainly those secreted by the adrenal cortex. Most of the metabolites of testosterone are biologically active. Testosterone and its activated metabolites are bound by receptor proteins in cells of sensitive organs and thence are taken into the nuclei where they bind to nucleoproteins. Testosterone promotes transcription or effects translation of stored genetic information as do other steroidal hormones [208]. The most obvious effects are on the organs of the male reproductive system, but many other organs are also sensitive to androgens. Testosterone increases muscle mass and promotes erythropoiesis. It is because of the latter property that testosterone and other androgens are sometimes used in the treatment of anemias. Androgenic activity is measured in animals by comparing the ratio of the increase in weight of the levator ani muscle to that of the seminal vesicle and ventral prostate compared to that of a standard compound such as testosterone. As with other steroids, the technique of radioimmunoassay permits measurements of very low concentrations of testosterone. Androgens begin to affect the male sex organs during fetal life. The testosterone derivative 5α-dihydrotestosterone (DHT) is believed to promote differentiation of the urogenital sinus (the

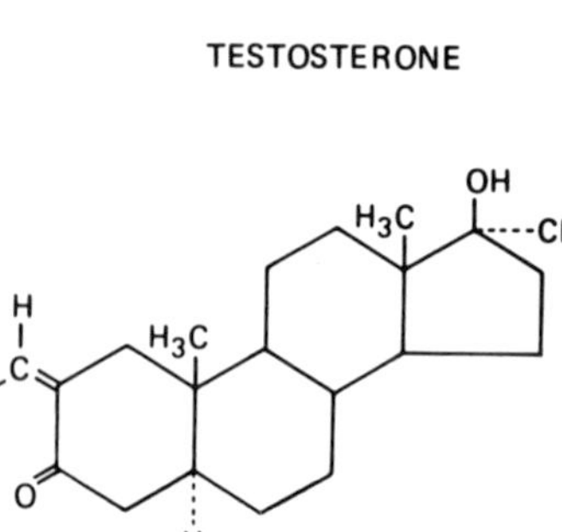

TESTOSTERONE 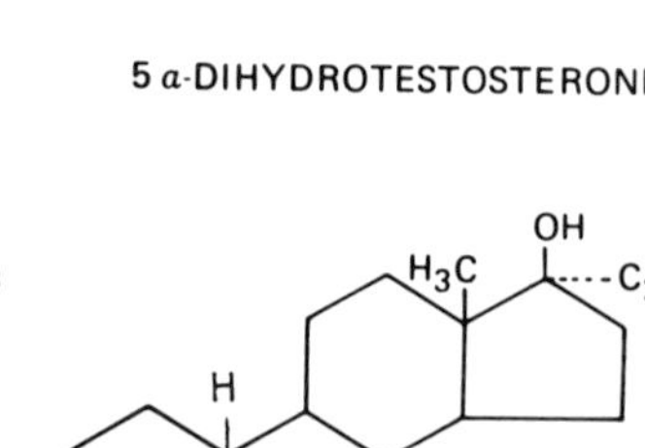   5 α-DIHYDROTESTOSTERONE (DHT)

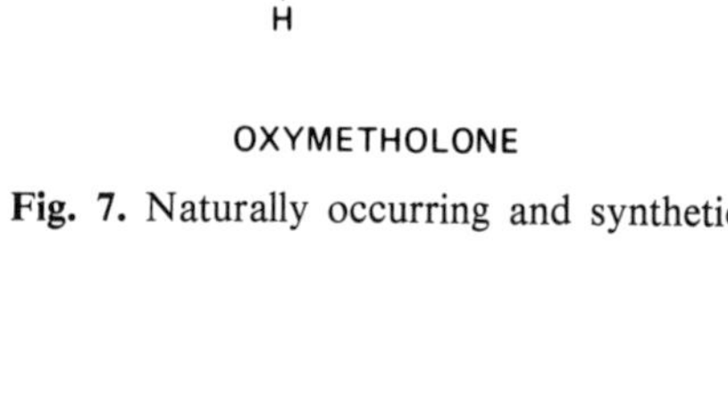

OXYMETHOLONE 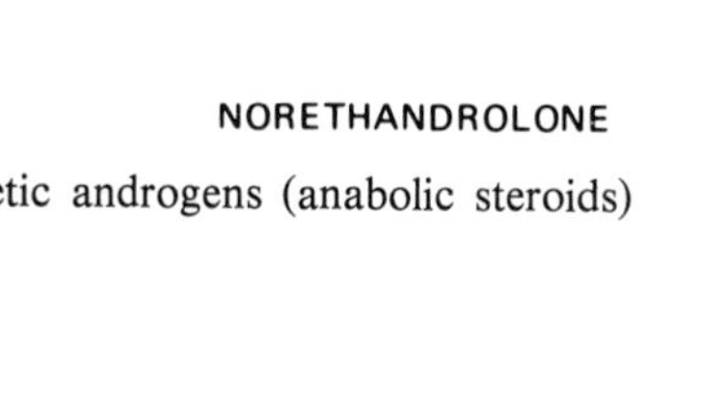   NORETHANDROLONE

Fig. 7. Naturally occurring and synthetic androgens (anabolic steroids)

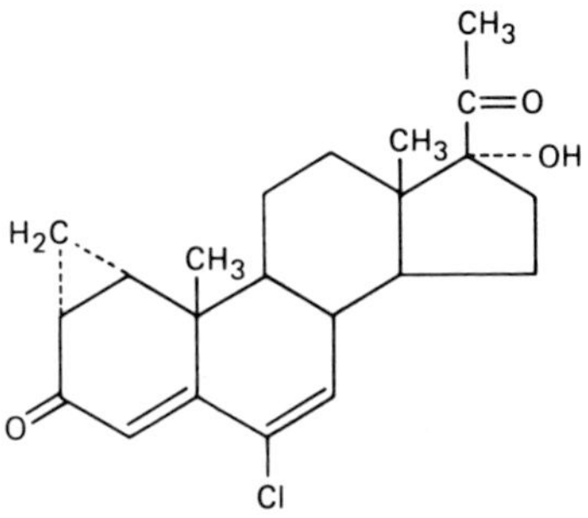

Fig. 8. The acetate of this synthetic compound is used as an anti-androgen

CYPROTERONE

anlage of the prostate) and the urogenital tubercle (the anlage of the external genitalia) whereas testosterone itself appears to be the critical hormone for differentiation of the wolffian duct system, which is the anlage of the epididymis, vas deferens, and seminal vesicles [208]. Compounds such as maternal estrogens that interfere with proper differentiation and growth of these target organs at critical stages of fetal life can cause malformations and possibly neoplasms. When given to pregnant rats, testosterone interveres with the development of genital organs of female fetuses.

Testosterone is produced commercially from cholesterol or diosgenin and is marketed mainly in the form of testosterone propionate and 17α-methyltestosterone. The so-called anabolic steroids take advantage of the fact that the myotropic and erythrogenic activity can be separated from the androgenic effects by structural rearrangements of the molecules (Fig. 7). Evidence of a *direct* role of endogenous androgens in induction of cancer is lacking, but there is presumptive evidence that both endogenous and exogenous androgens can be carcinogenic in some situations.

The potent anti-androgen *cyproterone acetate* (Fig. 8) developed during the 1960s as a progestin [155] is used in the treatment of male hypersexuality and deviationism, precocious puberty, prostate cancer, and female virilism despite a lack of adequate clinical trials and evidence of hepatocellular carcinogenicity in rats [46].

Other Hormones

Prolactin

There is no unequivocal evidence that prolactin is directly involved in neoplasia of the *human* mammary gland or other organ despite the fact that this polypeptide hormone, secreted by specialized cells of the anterior pituitary gland, participates in mammary gland carcinogenesis in mice [192]. Prolactin receptors have been demonstrated in DMBA-induced mammary gland tumors in Sprague-Dawley rats [35]. Increased levels of prolactin have been reported in sera of women from certain families with high frequencies of breast cancer [192], but results from other studies have been inconclusive. Prolactin secretion is regulated by a hypothalamic inhibitory neurohormone (prolactin inhibitory factor [PIF]). The secretion of prolactin can be inhibited by ergot alkaloids [192, 200] and L-dopa [192]. Chlorpromazine and other phenothiazines, reserpine, and tricyclic antidepressants block the synthesis, release, or action of PIF and thereby *increase* prolactin secretion [192], thus explaining the galactorrhea that sometimes occurs during the use of some of these drugs. This topic is discussed more fully in a subsequent paragraph. Interactions of prolactin and other endogenous and exogenous compounds are extremely complex and poorly understood.

Adrenal Cortical Steroids

The wide spectrum of metabolic activities of adrenal cortical steroids suggests that they may directly or indirectly influence the processes of neoplasia [202]. Clinical improvement of some patients with carcinoma of the breast following adrenalectomy indicates that the adrenal cortex can produce some cancer-promoting hormones, presumably estrogens or estrogen precursors. The adrenal cortex of both sexes produces estrogen precursor compounds that can be converted to estrogens in such tissues as body fat.
Untreated female mice of the NH strain develop estrogen-secreting adrenal cortical adenomas associated with early cessation of ovarian activity. Both male and female Bagg albino mice develop estrogen- and/or androgen-secreting adrenal cortical adenomas and carcinomas associated with declining but not total cessation of gonadal activity [175]. Sex-hormone secreting cortical adenomas can be induced in mice by castration [175].

Gonadotropic- and Hypothalamic-Releasing Hormones

There is very little evidence concerning the relation of these regulatory hormones to cancers of the organs that they control. Plasma gonadotropins increase in mice with neoplasms of spleen-implanted ovaries [175]. Estrogens induce neoplasms of the anterior pituitary in rats and mice of some strains [97]. Chorionic gonadotropic hormone is present in measurable amounts in the blood of some human patients with breast cancer, particularly those with metastatic disease [203]. Cells of certain neoplasms of the placenta and testes produce large amounts of gonadotropins, but these are not known to play a role in the *induction* of the neoplasms.

Hormone Receptors

The major steroid hormone receptors are proteins located in the cytoplasm and nuclei of cells, whereas the receptors for polypeptide hormones are located on the cell membrane [136]. Steroid receptors may be highly specific, as that for estradiol, or may exhibit a wide range of specificities, as for progesterone. A single cell may contain receptors for more than one steroid hormone. Steroid hormones enter the cytoplasm of responsive cells, probably by diffusion, attach to protein binders, and are transported into the nucleus where they bind with DNA and specific chromosomal proteins. There they alter patterns of gene expression and ultimately induce transcription of specific mRNAs. The remarkable specificity of receptor proteins for recognizing and distinguishing steroid hormones is illustrated by the fact that different tissues appear to contain distinct receptors for testosterone and dihydrotestosterone (DHT) [136]. The roles of hormones in modulating cellular activities is still only partly understood, but further elucidation of these mechanisms promises to be a fascinating episode in medical science.
Estrogen receptors are present in the breast and other organs of the female and male reproductive systems, the pituitary, liver, brain, myocardium, and other tissues. Estradiol receptors similar to those of uterine myometrium have been identified in the nuclei of myocardial fibers of the atria and auricles of male and female rats, but not in the myocytes of

the ventricles [196]. These receptors are also present in the media of arteries, the pericytes of capillaries, and in other locations. The significance of these findings is unclear, but such receptors could conceivable be involved in the pathogenesis of hypertension or other cardiovascular disease. Liver cytosol of at least four species (rats, mice, rabbits, and green monkeys) contains estrogen-binding macromolecules [49]. The binding of estradiol by the liver is relatively low compared to that by the uterus and is predominantly in the 4S rather than the 8S region, as shown by the uterine supernatant [49].

Estrogen receptors are present in interstitial cells of the testes of rats and mice. Interstitial cell tumors, some of which are estrogen dependent, can be induced in mice of susceptible strains such as C and BALB/c by implantation of DES [95, 187]. Interstitial cell tumors have been observed in a high percentage of *untreated* rats of some strains, e.g., F344 [193], but are not known to be associated with hyperestrogenism.

The main application of in vitro tests to determine the presence or absence of estrogen receptors in cancer cells is to predict response to hormonal therapy [129, 137, 161].

The concentration of uterine *progesterone receptors* in rats, mice, and hamsters varies during the estrous cycle and is controlled by estrogens. Estrogen induction of progesterone receptors appears to involve RNA and protein synthesis [51]. Clinical improvement of breast cancer patients following endocrine therapy correlates in as many as 90% of the cases with laboratory demonstration of receptors for both estrogen and progesterone [137].

Androgen receptors that can bind testosterone or 5α-dihydrotestosterone (DHT) have been found in many tissues of the rat. In addition to the male reproductive system (prostate, testes, epididymis, seminal vesicles), androgen receptors are present in kidney, sebaceous glands, submandibular glands, hair follicles, hypothalamus, pituitary, cerebral cortex, skeletal muscle, bone marrow, ovary, liver, lung, and heart [123]. Androgen receptors can be present in neoplastic cells from cancers of human mammary glands and androgen-dependent mammary tumors in mice [123], but their significance in the etiology of cancer is not known. Some human mammary gland carcinomas contain receptors for DHT, some contain both DHT and estradiol receptors, some have either one without the other, and some contain neither [167, 171]. So far, measurements of androgen receptors in cancers of the mammary gland, prostate, or other neoplasms have not permitted accurate predictions of clinical response to hormonal manipulations.

The so-called testicular feminization syndrome is believed to be a result of defective androgen receptors in cells of human males of the 46 XY karyotype [110]. The defect is present in the X chromosome, but the gonads of such individuals differentiate normally under the control of the Y chromosome. But because the gonads cannot respond to testosterone or its immediate derivative, 5α-dihydrotestosterone (DHT), these genotypic males develop as phenotypic females. The testicular feminization syndrome also occurs in rats and mice [110]. Defective receptors such as those that occur in this syndrome may play a role in carcinogenesis by rendering cells more susceptible to the action of carcinogens, but so far I know of no evidence to support such a hypothesis.

Specific receptors for *glucocorticoids* have been demonstrated in lymphocytes, including neoplastic cells from patients with leukemia [128]. The presence of such receptors on leukemic lymphocytes correlates to some degree with clinical response to steroid therapy. Despite the presence of these receptors in neoplastic cells, there is no evidence at this time that adrenocortical steroids participate in the etiology of leukemia or any other neoplasm.

As mentioned in an earlier paragraph, carcinogenic compounds may compete with hormones for receptor sites on cells and thus gain access to the genetic apparatus or other metabolic activity of the cell.

The Liver

Endogenous and exogenous steroids, nonsteroidal compounds, and a variety of other chemical compounds are metabolized in the liver by some of the same biochemical reactions. Similar enzymes activate, inactivate, conjugate, or otherwise alter the structures of many diverse chemicals including some that are carcinogenic. Endogenous or exogenous hormones can affect the activities of chemical carcinogens by several mechanisms or, conversely, their activities may be influenced by the presence of a variety or chemical compounds including many commonly used drugs [33]. Such compounds may interact with each other, induce, inactivate, or compete for available enzymes, potentiate or nullify reactivity of compounds, or otherwise affect the activities of a variety of similar or dissimilar compounds. For example, exogenous compounds such as phenobarbital and DDT, potent inducers of microsomal enzymes, increase the in vivo hydroxylation of progesterone, testosterone, and estradiol [3]. These compounds can competitively inhibit drug oxidation by hepatic microsomal mixed-function oxidative enzymes acting as alternative substrates. Testosterone promotes the hepatocellular neoplasia of some compounds, perhaps by inducing enzymes that activate carcinogens. There are many examples of interactions of chlorinated hydrocarbons with steroid hormones [112]. DDT derivatives can induce hepatic mixed-function oxidases, which stimulate the metabolism of steroid compounds, effectively decreasing the biologic activity of exogenous estrogens, androgens, and glucosteroids [112]. They can also combine with uterine estrogen receptors. Enzymes that conjugate estrogens with glucuronic acid are located in hepatic microsomes; their activity can be inhibited in rats by morphine, p-hydroxyamphetamine, and some metabolites of chlorpromazine [82]. Phenobarbital, 3-methylcholanthrene and 3,4-benzpyrene increase the conjugation of estrogens [82].

Rates and modes of metabolism as well as excretion of synthetic and naturally occurring hormones differ according to species, sex, and age [3]. The patterns of hepatic steroid metabolism in rats is the same in both sexes until puberty when the male liver begins to produce a pattern of C_{19} metabolites different from the juvenile and adult female patterns, an effect that can be abolished by castration within a few days after birth [24]. The "female pattern", determined by neonatal exposure of the liver to follicle-stimulating hormone (FSH) from the pituitary, consists of 5α-reduced, 3α- and 7α-hydroxylated steroids as the major C_{19} steroid metabolites, whereas at puberty, the male liver begins to form predominantly the 5β-reduced C_{19} steroids containing hydroxyl groups at positions 2α and β, 3α, 6β, and 16α. Castration prevents conversion to the male pattern [24].

Estrogens, progestins, and androgens appear to have different effects on the liver. Estrogens primarily affect protein synthesis in the rough ER (endoplasmic reticulum), whereas progestins and testosterone, the so-called anabolic steroids, mainly affect the smooth ER and drug-metabolizing enzymes [3]. Testosterone enhances nuclear RNA-synthesizing activity of hepatic cell nuclei in young male rats, an effect that is reduced by castration [123]. These activities can be restored in adult castrates by injection of DHT, but not in immature or senile male or in female rats because they cannot produce the DHT-binding receptors [123]. FSH but not luteinizing hormones (LH) may participate in the sex-dependent hydroxylase systems in the liver of rats [75].

Little is known about the capacity of the fetal liver to activate or inactivate carcinogenic or teratogenic chemical compounds. Some studies indicate that the fetal liver is capable of detoxifying and excreting some drugs early in gestation [177]. Experiments in which radiolabeled DES was given to pregnant mice indicated a 16-fold accumulation of [3_H] DES conjugates (primarily glucuronides) in the fetal liver, indicating activity of glucuronyltransferase in that organ. The placenta appears to restrict some of the movement of this synthetic hormone from mother to fetus [139].

Naturally occurring and some synthetic estrogens, $C 17\alpha$-alkyl substituted testosterones such as methyltestosterone, norethandrolone, and the 19-nortestosterone-derived progestins can, by mechanisms that are poorly understood, impair bile secretion in certain individuals as manifest by abnormalities in liver function tests or clinical cholestatic jaundice [3, 191]. Neither testosterone, its esters, nor progesterone appear to affect bile secretion [3]. Biliary excretion of hormones requires metabolic conjugation mainly with glucuronic acid or sulfates to form compounds of appropriate molecular weight and polarity. Incompletely understood variations in molecular configuration of steroids, such as the presence of an extra hydroxyl group, can affect biliary excretion.

Both endogenous and exogenous estrogens predispose to cholelithiasis and cholecystitis. These diseases are more frequent in women than men, in parous than in nonparous women, and in women taking exogenous estrogens [96]. Adenocarcinoma of the gallbladder and biliary ducts tend to occur more frequently in individuals with gallstones [47].

Some species variations in the patterns of biliary excretion and action of hydroxylating enzymes affect the metabolism of synthetic extrogens such as ethynylestradiol [85]. Genetic differences in individuals within human or animal populations probably account for some of the variations in reactivity. Differences in capacity for metabolizing bile pigments probably accounts for the recurrent cholestatic jaundice of pregnancy and that which occurs occasionally in women using oral contraceptives and may result from hereditary variations in the capacity to form drug-metabolizing enzymes or the sensitivity of the bile-processing functions of hepatocytes to steroids [3]. Individuals with the Crigler-Najjar syndrome and rats of the Gunn strain carry inherited defects in the ability to form bilirubin glucuronides [191].

One of the most spectacular effects of exogenous steroids on the liver is *peliosis hepatis,* an extreme dilatation of the sinusoids with formation of blood-filled cavities. This lesion has been observed in some patients receiving anabolic steroids, testosterone, and other androgens [19, 153] and in some women using oral contraceptives [153]. Hepatocellular neoplasms have also been observed in patients receiving synthetic anabolic steroids such as *oxymetholone* for treatment of aplastic anemia, particularly the hereditary Fanconi's type [52] (Table 3) (see ISHAK, this monograph). Athletes of both sexes sometimes use these materials to increase muscle mass, a practice that has been discouraged by the medical profession [206]. So far, I am not aware of instances of peliosis hepatis or hepatocellular neoplasms that could be attributed to this nonmedical use of these hormones. It may be that a healthy person can metabolize these compounds without pathologic effects, but it would not be surprising if some of these men and women develop disturbances in liver function and possibly neoplasms.

Reports of hepatocellular neoplasms in patients receiving anabolic steroids and other androgens for replacement or treatment of anemia or other diseases have also been received with skepticism by some who insist that these proliferative lesions are not neoplasms because they have rarely been observed to metastasize outside the liver and in some instances have regressed after cessation of therapy (see ISHAK, this monograph). Androgens have long been known to promote hepatocellular carcinogenicity of other compounds such as azo dyes when given to laboratory animals [126]. It may be that anabolic steroids promote neoplasia induced by other carcinogens. The fact that these hormones contribute in any way to the processs of neoplasia, regardless of the mechanism, indicates a need for caution in their use, particularly for such frivolous and questionable purposes as muscle-building. Their use in grave diseases such as aplastic anemias is a different matter, although evidence of a favorable influence in these diseases has not been subjected to rigorous clinical trials. Androgens used in the treatment of endometriosis or breast cancer have not yet been implicated in neoplasms of the liver or other organs. Women receiving such compounds for any purpose, however, should remain under careful surveillance for long periods of time after the therapy is completed.

The controversies about the carcinogenic hazards of steroids in oral contraceptives have centered on the pathologic interpretations of the hepatocellular lesions and the appropriateness of tests in animals for correctly predicting carcinogenicity in man. As it has turned out, the proliferative lesions in livers of rats given oral contraceptive steroids did correctly predict that similar lesions might occur in women and should have received more attention when first noted in the early 1960s [29, 178]. Changes ranging from hyperplasia to hepatocellular carcinoma were reported in 13% of rats receiving a combination of ethynylestradiol and norethindrone acetate, in 32% of male rats receiving norethynodrel, in 23% of those receiving a combination of mestranol and norethisterone and in 17% given ethynylestradiol. Not until 1973, when hepatocellular neoplasms were reported in women using these drugs, did reports of similar neoplasms in test animals receive attention. The issue is complicated because of difficulties in predicting the behavior of hepatocellular neoplasms by histopathologic criteria alone. As discussed more fully in this monograph by ISHAK, most hepatocellular neoplasms in women using oral contraceptives have, by conventional biologic and histologic criteria, proved to be benign, but a worrisome few have behaved as malignant neoplasms with invasion and metastases. Furthermore some histologically benign tumors have killed their hosts by rupture and subsequent hemorrhage. Observations of hepatocellular neoplasms in rats and mice exposed to a variety of carcinogens have indicated no precise boundary between "benign" and "malignant" and the lack of such boundaries should counter any complacent attitudes regarding the long-term effects of these products in women.

Hormones in Relation to Cancers of Specific Sites

The Breast

Neoplasia of human and animal mammary glands is critically dependent on stimulation by hormones at some stage in development regardless of the other factors involved in the etiology. The interplay of hormones, viruses, and genetic factors in mammary gland carcinogenesis in mice has been described at length in other publications [175] and will not be repeated here. Despite the abundance of information about the roles of hormones in mammary carcinogenesis in animals, the roles of hormones secreted by ovaries, pituitary, adrenals, or other tissues in induction and promotion of the common ductal carcinoma of the *human* female breast remains controversial although isolated bits of information suggest that an underlying abnormality in the production or metabolism of one or more hormones may be involved [107].

The most convincing arguments supporting a role of *endogenous* hormones in the etiology of human breast cancer are:

1. The rarity of breast cancer prior to puberty;
2. The protection afforded by castration at young ages [134] (also in dogs, mice, and rats);
3. The favorable clinical response of many breast cancers to ablation of the ovaries, adrenals, or to treatment with androgens or estrogens;

4. The relative protective effects of pregnancy (by contrast, mammary gland carcinomas of mice of some strains are more frequent in breeders than in virgins) [175];
5. The induction of carcinomas in males by exogenous estrogens;
6. Epidemiologic associations of cancer of the breast with other estrogen-dependent cancers such as those of the endometrium; and
7. The increased risk of mammary gland cancers in women receiving replacement estrogens.

As shown in Table 1, the suspicion that pregnancy offered protection against breast cancer dates back to 1713 [62]. Later studies indicated that this protective effect is only relative and the first pregnancy must be full-term and must occur before the age of 30 years [134]. Nevertheless, the majority of breast cancer patients are normal, "feminine", multiparous women. Lactation per se does not appear to be a dominant protective characteristic.

As mentioned under the discussion of hormone receptors, the clinical response of breast cancer to oophorectomy, adrenalectomy, or treatment with exogenous hormones cannot always be predicted from the presence or absence of hormone receptors. Hormone dependency appears to become "lost" in stages during the progression of the cancers to full autonomy. The basis for the favorable responses of some older women with breast cancer to exogenous estrogen is not known, but it may involve a repression of pituitary hormones or other mechanisms.

Thus far the many attempts to demonstrate differences in production or metabolism of endogenous hormones that would predict which women are most likely to develop breast cancer have failed to reveal a "clear cut or comprehensible" pattern [107]. It is difficult to reconcile all the data on the frequencies of hormone-related cancers in world populations with ideas that genetic differences in metabolism of estrogens and other hormones are the major etiologic determinants. Genetic differences cannot explain why immigrants from a low-risk country such as Japan develop breast cancer at a rate similar to other Americans within a few years of migration, both in the immigrants themselves and in their first generation offspring [26]. This increased risk is similar to that for cancers of the prostate, endometrium, ovary, and colon [27, 77]. Thus, despite a role of hormones in the etiology of most of these cancers, the major determinants must be sought in the environment.

Diet is an obvious environmental influence that undergoes pronounced changes during Americanization and has been blamed for the major epithelial cancers, except for those of the lung, in the United States and Europe. Diets high in meat and animal fat are suspected of playing a role in the etiology of many cancers that occur in men and women past middle age although solid evidence supporting this hypothesis is scant. Estrogens, such as estradiol, estrone, and 17-methoxyestradiol, can be produced in vitro by intestinal bacteria from cholestenone, a bacterial metabolite of cholesterol, and other compounds in feces [91]. The bacteria are lecithinase-negative *Clostridia,* a minor component of normal intestinal flora. People consuming diets high in fat would be expected to produce greater quantities of such abnormal steroids, but there is no evidence that these reactions occur in vivo or that such steroids are carcinogenic.

In addition to endogenous hormones, human and animal mammary glands are exposed to a large number of exogenous compounds for which there is actual or presumptive evidence of estrogenic activity. These include not only pharmaceutical preparations but hormonomimetic compounds in food and miscellaneous compounds of industrial origin that widely contaminate the environment.

Pharmaceutical preparations are obvious sources for prolonged exposure of large numbers of women to potent estrogens. A 1976 report indicates that women who use conjugated estrogens for replacement are at greater risk of developing breast cancer than nonusers [93].

A study by FECHNER [53], however, indicated that breast cancers in women using conjugated estrogens do not differ in histopathologic characteristics from those that occur in non-users.

So far an increase in breast cancer has not occurred in users of oral contraceptives and most studies have indicated a *decrease* in frequency of benign disease in users [54] (see HILLIARD and NORRIS, this monograph). There has been no excess of mammary gland neoplasms in animals, including monkeys, receiving oral contraceptives long term [54] except for the controversial lesions in beagles discussed by CASEY et al. (this monograph). Although these proliferative lesions have no direct counterpart in women, the experiences with extrogen-induced neoplasms of the vagina and liver in young women indicate that any type of *proliferative* lesion in test animals should be regarded as warnings and are not to be dismissed lightly. It is not possible to "prove" safety of any compound, but those that induce any type of growth disturbance are the most obvious candidates for intensive studies of possible carcinogenicity.

Hormones other than estrogens and progestins that may participate in the etiology of neoplasms of mammary glands in experimental animals include *prolactin* (discussed in a previous section), *thyrotropin-releasing hormone* [30], and possibly others. *Insulin* and *cortisol* are involved in milk protein formation of normal mammary glands and insulin has been suggested to play a role in mammary gland carcinogenesis [129]. Hormones from the thyroid and thymus glands may also play a role in the etiology of cancer of the mammary glands, but evidence of such possible associations is scant at the present time. As discussed earlier, *prolactin* has not yet been shown to participate in the induction of *human* breast cancer. The role of *pituitary gonadotropins* is also unclear. The fact that breast cancer is most frequent after the menopause suggests that the increased levels of luteinizing hormone (LH) and follicle-stimulating hormone (FSH) in response to the decreasing levels of endogenous estrogens from the involuting ovaries may play a role in the etiology of breast cancer at ages past 55. Breast cancer in older women, in contrast to that in younger women, frequently improves following treatment with estrogens. If pituitary gonadotropins are involved in the induction of breast cancer in older women, it is possible that exogenous estrogens, if used in doses only sufficient to control the excessive production of pituitary gonadotropins, might, in some women, actually *prevent* rather than induce breast cancer. Evidence for a role of pituitary gonadotropins in the etiology of breast cancer in the human *male* is suggested by the report of a man who developed breast cancer 30 years after bilateral mumps orchitis and subsequent testicular atrophy [156] as well as the increased risk of breast cancer in men with Klinefelter's syndrome. Males with this syndrome, usually with a 47 XXY genotype, characteristically have atrophy of the seminiferous tubules and gynecomastia, which is associated with an increased excretion of pituitary gonadotropins [73, 150].

The male mammary gland is susceptible to induction of cancer by *exogenous* estrogens. More than 40 years ago, LACASSAGNE induced mammary gland cancers in male *mice* by injecting estrone [117]. Exogenous estrogens are believed to have caused bilateral breast carcinomas in two *human* male transsexuals who received estrogens (the type of preparation was not reported) following surgical castration [199]. Several men who received DES for treatment of carcinoma of the prostate developed carcinomas in their breasts [34]. Most of these are now believed to be metastases from the prostate [149] rather than primary breast cancers. The breast is ordinarily an unusual site for metastases from any cancer in men and women, but perhaps the explanation for this unusual complication in men receiving DES for prostate cancer might be that the mammary tissue was excessively stimulated by the DES and thus made more receptive to metastases.

That endogenous estrogens may be involved in the etiology of cancer of the male breast is indicated by reports of abnormally high levels of urinary estrogens in men with breast cancer [37, 50, 213]. Men with Klinefelter's syndrome have a frequency of breast cancer approaching that of women [74, 99, 162], although this syndrome accounts for only about 3% of all male breast cancers.

A relationship between breast cancer and *gynecomastia* is indicated by the higher frequency of cancers in breasts of men with gynecomastia than in those without it. For example, a history of gynecomastia was recorded in 10 of 265 men with primary breast cancer in the records of the Danish Tumor Registry [179]. Gynecomastia should not be regarded as a precancerous lesion because the majority of male breast cancers do not originate in breasts exhibiting gynecomastia and cancer has rarely, if ever, been observed to originate in hyperplastic epithelium of classic gynecomastia, a distinct histopathologic entity. Care must be taken in interpreting reports of a relationship between cancer and gynecomastia because other hyperplastic lesions of the male breast can be confused with gynecomastia.

The cause of gynecomastia is not known in most instances. It is fairly common in men with cirrhosis and has been attributed to hyperestrogenism resulting from the failure of the damaged liver in this disease to remove estrogens, but other mechanisms may be involved. Hyperplastic lesions including gynecomastia may occur following occupational exposure to estrogens. Enlargement of one or both breasts was observed in 20 of 38 men engaged in the manufacture of DES in one plant [56]. Histopathologic examinations of several surgically excised lesions from these men indicated hyperplasia or gynecomastia. Most of these lesions regressed after cessation of exposure. There were no cancers observed in these men at the time of the report in 1945, but now that more than 30 years have passed an effort should be made to locate these men for study since they would appear to be at unusual risk for cancer. Subsequent reports have related hyperplastic lesions of the male breast to exposure to estrogens during commercial synthesis. Hyperestrogenism has been observed in male and female children of women engaged in the manufacture of estrogens, mainly DES, which were traced to contamination of the home environment by materials carried on the clothing [25]. WATROUS and OLSEN [207] reviewed all the literature referring to signs of hyperestrogenism in both male and female factory workers, and in some instances their children, in several countries of the world due to exposure to various synthetic and naturally occurring estrogens during commercial production. He also described the protective procedures adopted in some plants in the United States to protect workers from effects of such exposure[1].

The Ovary

Hormonal stimulation plays an uncertain role in the etiology of carcinoma of the human ovary [127]. As with cancer of the breast and endometrium, several reports indicate that nulliparous women are at greater risk of cancer of the ovary than those who have borne children [86, 101]. Variations in the incidence of epithelial cancers of the human ovary are comparable worldwide to those of breast, endometrium, prostate, and colon; increases in rates following migration from low- to high-risk countries suggest, as with these other cancers, the influence of external factors such as diet. A recent preliminary report [94] suggests that

---

1 In 1977 an American manufacturer of DES was fined $ 34,000 by the U.S. Occupational Safety and Health Administration (OSHA) following development of breast enlargements and impotence in 9 of 17 workers exposed to DES (*The Washington Post*, June 18, 1977).

women who use DES for replacement in addition to conjugated estrogens may be at a greater risk of ovary cancer than other women. Hypersecretion of hormones from the anterior pituitary induces certain types of neoplasms in the ovaries of mice [175], but this phenomenon is not known to occur in women with this frequent form of cancer.

The Endometrium

The uterine endometrium is influenced by both endogenous and exogenous estrogens. Hyperplasia of the endometrial glands is associated with steroid-secreting stromal neoplasms of the ovary in women and in rats [193]. The relation of simple and atypical hyperplasia to adenocarcinoma in women is still uncertain, but many pathologists believe that the markedly atypical hyperplasia may be a precursor to adenocarcinoma in some women; they disagree about the precise criteria for distinguishing "atypical adenomatous hyperplasia" from adeno-carcinoma [88]. A definite transition from adenomatous hyperplasia to invasive adenocarci-noma can be seen in the rat [193]. Both atypical hyperplasias and adenocarcinomas are more frequent than expected in women taking exogenous estrogens, mainly conjugated equine preparations [189, 212]. An increased risk of endometrial adenocarcinoma is also observed in women using the sequential type of oral contraceptive [131, 188] (see HILLIARD and NORRIS, this monograph), in women with gonadal dysgenesis treated with replacement hormones [36], and in women with breast cancer who receive estrogens, predominantly nonsteroidal types such as DES [92].

As in breast cancer patients, attempts to demonstrate specific underlying abnormalities in production or utilization of hormones in patients with this cancer have yielded little usable information for identifying women at highest risk. Obesity, hypertension, and a diabetic pattern of glucose tolerance are unusually frequent in women with endometrial carcinoma [81]. Such women appear to have underlying abnormalities in the endocrine system. Obesity is believed to contribute to a "hyperestrogenic" state because excessive amounts of estrone can be produced from adrenal or ovarian androstenedione in body fat. The relative deficiency of progesterone cannot counteract the stimulatory effects of estrone on the endometrium in women with involuting ovaries.

Carcinoma of the endometrium is most frequent worldwide in populations with the highest frequencies of cancers of the breast, ovary, and colon and shares with these a higher frequency in nulliparous as compared to multiparous women. Indeed, carcinoma of the endometrium is more likely to develop in women with a previous carcinoma of the breast [133, 183] and, conversely, women with carcinoma of the endometrium are unusually susceptible to subse-quent primary cancers of the breast and ovary [183]. Women treated for carcinoma of the breast with estrogens are especially prone to adenocarcinoma of the endometrium [92].

Adenocarcinoma of the endometrium is infrequent in most animals except in rabbits of some strains [72, 106] and cattle [106, 145]. Adenocarcinoma, preceded by cystic hyperplasia, is one of the most frequent neoplasms of untreated domestic rabbits. GREENE observed that adenocarcinoma of the uterus almost invariably occurred in rabbits that survived toxemia of pregnancy and suggested that it might result from hyperestrogenism because of damage to the liver [72]. Occasionally rabbits with endometrial adenocarcinoma also developed squamous cell carcinoma of the vagina but not the cervix [72]. Both cystic hyperplasia and adenocarci-noma of the endometrium were reported in rabbits given DES, but too few animals were used to be certain of the inductive effects of the hormone [142]. Adenocarcinoma of the mammary gland and abnormalities of other endocrine organs were also noted in rabbits in GREENE's laboratory.

The Cervix

Epidemiologic evidence suggests that viruses and/or other environmental factors play a major role in the etiology of this frequent cancer, the majority of which are squamous cell carcinomas. Evidence also points to the possible role of hormonal stimulation. The host susceptibility factors appear to be "opposite" those of cancers of the breast and endometrium, i.e., the disease is almost entirely limited to parous women. Desipite evidence that cancer of the cervix may be an infectious disease spread by sexual intercourse, the role of viruses is uncertain. One study indicated that more women of ages 20—50 years with this neoplasm had abnormalities of the menstrual cycles and lower levels of 13 urinary steroids than patients with breast cancer, thus suggesting some abnormality originating in the pituitary hypothalamic regulatory system [109].

It is not known if *exogenous* estrogens play a significant role in the etiology of primary carcinoma of the human cervix, but several estrogens have induced or promoted neoplasms in the cervix of mice. Studies attempting to link precancerous lesions and carcinomas of the human cervix to the use of oral contraceptives have yielded equivocal results (see HILLIARD and NORRIS, this monograph). I know of no evidence that *replacement* estrogens are involved in neoplasia of the human cervix, but case control studies of older women with invasive carcinomas should include questions about experience with these compounds.

Primary neoplasms of the cervix are rare in untreated animals. Squamous cell carcinoma of the cervix can be induced in mice by several estrogens, including DES (see DUNN, this monograph). DES promotes the development of squamous cell carcinoma of the mouse cervix induced by the direct application of 3-methylcholanthrene [151] whereas *castration* retards the process [152]. Among the many reports of attempts using various techniques to induce cancer of the cervix in animals is the 1935 paper by OVERHOLSER and ALLEN [166] describing "atypical growths" in the epithelium of the cervix of rhesus monkeys given estrogens S.C. and subjected to mechanical trauma directly on the cervix. Both descriptions and illustrations indicate epidermidalization of cervical glands, but the other changes described in the paper are difficult to evaluate; the authors did not claim to have induced invasive neoplasms.

The Vagina

The human vagina is an infrequent site for primary neoplasms. Most that do occur are of three distinctive histologic types:
1. squamous cell carcinoma;
2. mixed Müllerian tumors [88]; and
3. adenocarcinoma.

Squamous cell carcinoma is the most frequent type of vaginal cancer. It occurs mainly in older women and is most frequently located on the posterior wall in the upper two-thirds of the vagina. This form of cancer is usually highly invasive and rapidly fatal (Fig. 9). No precancerous lesions or associated abnormal hormonal stimulations are known to be involved in the etiology. Women with this form of cancer should be questioned about their experiences with exogenous estrogens since estrogens definitely induce squamous cell carcinomas in the vagina in old mice.

The *mixed Müllerian tumor* (botryoid sarcoma) is more likely to originate in the vagina in infants and young children, but the uterus is the more frequent site in adults. This neoplasm, which is very undifferentiated, originates in cells of the mucosal stroma and is composed of variable proportions of sarcomatous and carcinomatous elements. Hormonal stimulation is not known to play a role in the etiology, but the occurrence of this neoplasm in infants suggests that prenatal exposure to carcinogens may be a factor.

Adenocarcinoma originating in the vagina was a rare neoplasm prior to reports of clear-cell adenocarcinomas associated with prenatal exposure to DES (see KURMAN, this monograph).

In animals primary neoplasms of the vagina are rare. Although they are occasionally observed in old untreated mice, particularly those of an inbred line derived from the Pybus-Miller stock [65], most reports of the murine neoplasm have been associated with exposure to exogenous estrogens (Table 5). These experiments were performed under widely varying conditions. Many different estrogen preparations were given by different routes and dosage schedules. Mice of strains differing in susceptibility were maintained for varying periods of time, often less than 1 year. Several investigators, however, did maintain their animals for more than 2 years; they performed careful post-mortem dissections and histopathologic examinations, and some attempts were made to transplant the cervicovaginal lesions. The descriptions and photographs in many of these papers clearly indicate pathologic processes similar to those described and illustrated by DUNN in 1963 [43, 44] and reproduced in this monograph. Although the succession of changes from hyperplasia to neoplasia resulted in invasive carcinoma in only a small percent of exposed animals in all of the reports, a squamous cell carcinoma in one C3H mouse in GARDNER's experiments extended through the walls of the cervix, vagina, rectum, and adjacent structures of the pelvis and lumbar lymph

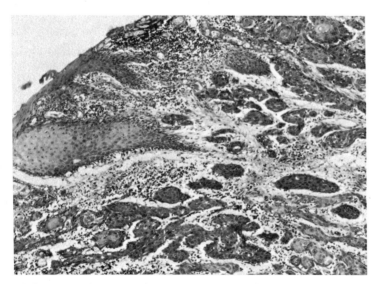

Fig. 9. Human vagina, squamous cell carcinoma. Note the resemblance of this neoplasm to DES-induced squamous cell carcinomas of the mouse vagina illustrated by DUNN (this monograph). H & E, × 80

nodes and proved to be transplantable through three generations [64]. Comparable neoplasms were not observed in any of the 104 controls of the same strains, some untreated, and some treated with the sesame oil vehicle with and without cholesterol or cholesterol benzoate [64]. GARDNER consistently noted that the invasive vaginocervical lesions developed only in mice that survived 300–400 days. Many C3H and CBA mice developed mammary gland cancers at young ages and did not survive long enough to develop vaginocervical neoplasms. Invasive lesions of cervix and vagina, as mentioned before, are infrequent in untreated mice of most strains.

BERN et al. [14, 102] also induced a similar sequence of pathologic changes in the cervix and vagina of mice with estrogens and progesterone. Some of these were successfully transplanted. FORSBERG [59] observed changes similar to those described by DUNN and GREEN [44] in the vagina and cervix of mice of the NMRI strain given DES and estradiol-17β as newborns. The mice developed ovary-dependent persistent vaginal cornification and focal replacement of squamous epithelium by columnar epithelium. Later the epithelium formed "glandular" downgrowths into the stroma, in some cases penetrating as far as the mesothelial surface. FORSBERG has published extensive descriptions of the embryologic development of the uterus and vagina in the human as well as in the mouse, rat, and other animals [57]. He suggested that adenosis of the human vagina may originate in Müllerian-derived columnar epithelium that has failed to undergo the normal transition to squamous epithelium because of altered hormonal environment during critical stages, such as exposure to DES or other hormones in utero [58]. The murine lesions described to date are different from the human lesions, possibly because of differences in the embryologic development in the two species. In mice, the demarcation of the squamous epithelium covering the uterine cervix and vagina is indefinite at the junction, whereas that of the human cervix with its characteristic cervical glands, absent in the mouse, is sharply demarcated and abruptly changes to that lining the vagina.

NOMURA and KANZAKI [160] found no proliferative lesions of the vagina-cervix in offspring of mice of the CR/Jcl strain given a single S.C. injection of DES during pregnancy or in mice of the same strain injected 12 h or 21 days after birth; however, all mice were killed 12 months after birth or treatment and there was probably not time for proliferative changes to occur.

Female *hamsters* exposed as fetuses to DES given by intragastric tube to their mothers during pregnancy developed endometrial hyperplasia and one developed endometrial adenocarcinoma. Other animals developed a variety of lesions including endocervical polyps and squamous cell papillomas of the cervix and vagina; one mouse had a mixed mesenchymal tumor of the cervix [176]. Males developed spermatic granulomas of the epididymis; one developed an adenoma of Cowper's glands and another a leiomyosarcoma of the seminal vesicles. A relationship between all these diverse lesions and the hormonal stimulation is uncertain. A 1978 WHO publication lists additional ongoing experiments designed to test effects of DES and other estrogens on fetal hamsters [209].

Few reports in the literature describe effects of estrogens on the genitalia of *rats*. SNELL (personal communication) exposed fetal rats of two strains (SD/N and F344/N) to DES dissolved in cottonseed oil in total doses up to 0.40 mg (strain designations are those of FESTING and STAATS [55]). Pregnant females received DES or cottonseed oil alone by stomach tube daily for 2, 3, or 4 days on gestation days 12–16. It was difficult to achieve a dose tolerated by the rats and many aborted during the initial phases of the study. Seventy-three offspring (30 males and 43 females) so exposed survived 20 months or more. At necropsy, none had grossly visible abnormalities of genitalia or other systems that could be

Table 5. Selected reports of proliferative lesions of vagina and cervix of mice receiving estrogens[a]

	Year	Strain[b]		Survival	Pathologic lesions
Suntzeff et al. [197]	1938	A, C57, D, C3H, CBA, New Buffalo, Old Buffalo	Theelin or theelol[c] injected at regular intervals. Some animals also received extracts from pituitary and/or lutein hormone	Up to 25 months	Invasive, proliferative lesions of epithelium of vagina and/or cervix observed in 25 of 234 surviving treated animals and in 1 of 128 untreated controls
Gardner and Allen [64]	1939	C3H, CBA, C$_{12}$I, A, N, JK, C57, F	Estradiol benzoate, equilin, equilenin benzoate, estradiol benzoate, estradiol dipropionate, or stilbestrol in sesame oil injected S.C. weekly. A few mice received progesterone or testosterone simultaneously	Variable. Some survived more than 1 year	Proliferative lesions of vagina-cervix with varying degrees of invasiveness in 27 of 183 treated mice. Three were classified squamous cell carcinomas. One was transplantable through three generations. No comparable lesions in any of the 104 controls, untreated or given sesame oil alone or with cholesterol or cholesterol benzoate
Murphy [151]	1961	C3Hf/He, A/He	DES, 5 mg of 10% or 33% in cholesterol, implanted S.C., interscapular, at 1.5–4 months of age	Many survived more than 1 year	Squamous cell carcinomas of cervix-vagina in 6 of 84 mice receiving DES alone. There were none in untreated controls. (Other mice received 3-methylcholanthrene applied directly to the cervix with and without DES)

attributed to DES. Examination of histologic material from these rats has not been completed, but slides are on file at the National Cancer Institute's Registry of Experimental Cancers and can be examined there. Rats of the McCollum strain did not develop neoplasms of the vagina or cervix following long-term feeding of ethynylestradiol, with and without megestrol acetate [138].

	Year	Strain	Treatment	Observation	Results
Dunn and Green [44]	1963	BALB/c, C3H/f	DES, 0.1 ml of a 2% suspension in saline injected S.C. on back within 24 h of birth	13–26 months	Cancers or precancers of vagina/cervix in 17 of 30 female mice surviving more than 13 months. Two were transplantable. One untreated C3H/f mouse with a granulosa cell tumor of the overy and evidence of continuous estrogen stimulation developed a carcinoma of the vagina near the vaginal orifice
Kimura and Nandi [105]	1967	BALB/cCrgl	Estradiol-17 β or testosterone, 0.1, 5 or 25 µg/day in 5% gum arabic in distilled water injected on 5 consecutive days beginning within 24 h after birth. Approximately one-half were ovariectomized at age 110–120 days	Killed at ages 15–17 months	Vaginal epithelial cornification, parakeratosis, stromal down-growths of epithelium, in all 46 intact mice receiving the estrogen. Hyperplastic lesions "resembling epidermoid carcinomas" developed in vagina or cervix of 13 of 16 mice receiving the highest dose. The lesions were less severe in ovariectomized mice. Some mice receiving testosterone alone developed similar hyperplastic lesions
Dunn [43]	1969	BALB/c	Enovid (mestranol and norethynodrel) in Metrecal (oral) (estimated 10–12.5 µg/day/mouse)	Killed at 518–721 days	"Early cancer or infiltrating cancer" observed in 6 of 6 mice receiving Enovid continuously from age 105 days and in two offspring of a pregnant mouse that received Enovid and which also received Enovid from weaning at age 37 days. No similar lesions in 42 untreated female BALB/c mice ages 24–30 months autopsied during the same period

Despite the transplantability and other evidence of malignant behavior, the vagina-cervix neoplasms of mice induced by exogenous estrogens is discounted by some investigators who require histologic identity between the human and murine lesions. The low frequency of these neoplasms in exposed mice is also cited by these critics as evidence against the carcinogenicity of estrogens. Yet experience with other classes of chemical carcinogens has indicated many

Table 5. (continued)

		Strain[b]		Survival	Pathologic lesions
Heston et al. [90]	1973	BALB/cHe, C3H/He, C3HfB/He, A/He, C57B1/He	Enovid in pellets (oral) at 3 dose levels, estimated 10, 20, and 40 µg/day	Ages given as averages. The oldest survivors of treated mice were BALB/c with average age at death 655 days	"Epithelial lesions" of cervix and vagina in 64 of 694 treated and 58 of 694 controls
Jones and Bern [102]	1977	BALB/cfC3H/ Crgl	17β-estradiol and/or progesterone in sesame oil, 5 or 20 µg, injected daily, S.C. beginning 36 h after birth. Approximately one-half were ovariectomized on day 40	Killed at onset of mammary neoplasms or 52 weeks	Hyperplastic lesions (cornification, parakeratosis, basal cell downgrowth) of cervix/ vagina in all mice except those receiving the lowest dose of estrogen and progesterone which were ovariectomized

[a] Some mice received progestins or other compounds simultaneously.
[b] Strain designations are those given by author.
[c] Names of hormone preparations are those given by author; see Fig. 2.

examples of differences between species in location and histopathologic characteristics of neoplasms induced by the same compound.

Neoplasms and malformations of the genitalia following intrauterine exposure to DES emphasize the role of the placenta and fetal tissues in the metabolism of toxic and carcinogenic chemical compounds. Endogenous and exogenous hormones and many other compounds

Table 6. Reports of abnormalities of the male genital system of animals induced by DES

		Age			
Shimkin and Grady [186]	1941	2 months at beginning of experiment	Oral (in food)	Mice: strain C3H[a]	Scrotal herniation, decreased spermatogenesis
Shimkin et al. [187]	1941	6 weeks at beginning of experiment	S.C. (cholesterol pellets)	Mice: strain C[a]	Interstitial cell tumors of testes
Dunn and Green [44]	1963	Newborn	S.C.	Mice: strains BALB/c and C3Hf[a]	Epididymal cysts
McLachlan et al. [140]	1975	In utero	S.C.	Mice: strain CD-1	Cryptorchidism, hypoplasia, and fibrosis of retained testes, epididymal cysts
Rustia and Shubik [176]	1976	In utero	Intragastric	Hamsters	Spermatic granulomas of epididymis
Nomura and Kanzaki [160]	1977	In utero	S.C.	Mice: strain ICR/Jcl	Cryptorchidism and hypotrophic testes

[a] Strain designations are those given by author.

in the maternal circulation cross the placenta and enter the fetal circulation. The placenta, in conjunction with the fetal and maternal livers and adrenals — the so-called fetoplacental unit — produces many biologically active compounds including estrogens, progesterone, androgens, corticosteroids, human chorionic gonadotropin (HCG), and human placental lactogen [39, 97]. Estrogens, mainly *estriol*, increase to very high levels in both mother and fetus during gestation. Some are synthesized by the placenta and fetal liver from dehydroepiandrosterone secreted by the fetal adrenal and some are transferred to the fetus from the maternal circulation, mostly in the unconjugated state [97]. Low levels of maternal estriol, associated with malfunction of the fetoplacental unit, and fetal adrenal hypoplasia have been noted to correlate with high fetal mortality, intrauterine growth retardation, and major fetal malformations, mainly anencephaly [38], Down's syndrome [103], and other syndromes associated with chromosome abnormalities [168]. The placenta produces most of the progesterone during the second and third trimesters [39]. Certain synthetic progestins cause masculinization of the fetus [200], but there is no evidence that *endogenous* progesterone has similar effects. Exposure to exogenous estrogens and progesterones during fetal life increases the likelihood of congenital anomalies of the heart [84]. Such exposure may also result in neoplasms of nongenital organs as illustrated by the single case report of a rare type of hepatocellular neoplasm (hepatoblastoma) in a 7-month-old male infant whose mother had taken a progestin-only contraceptive, 18-methylnorethisterone (Norgestrel, Wyeth), 30 μg daily during the first 3 months of pregnancy [165].

Both the placenta and fetal liver synthesize drug-metabolizing enzymes [141]. As early as the 14th week, the human fetal liver shows some drug-metabolizing activity. During gestation the levels reach approximately one-third that of the adult liver [68, 141]. The human fetal liver contains more cytochrome P450 enzymes and is capable of more microsomal activity than that of most laboratory animals [141]. Cytochrome P450 enzymes are very low in the fetuses of rats, guinea pigs, rabbits, and hamsters; their presence in rabbit fetuses can be demonstrated by very sensitive methods at 2—10 days before birth [68]. The activities of these enzymes increase to adult levels within 3—8 weeks after birth and parallel the development of the liver endoplasmic reticulum [68]. Liver microsomes from human fetuses can metabolize substances as testosterone, ethylmorphine, chlorpromazine, hexobarbital, and others [68]. The human fetal liver and other tissues can also convert androstenedione to estrone [180].

Male mice, in response to intrauterine or neonatal exposure to DES (Table 6), develop malformations of the sexual organs and interstitial neoplasms of the testes [187]. So far, I am unaware of testicular neoplasms developing in cryptorchid testes of mice, but the human cryptorchid testis is unusually susceptible to germ cell neoplasms.

The *human male* fetus is also susceptible to damage to genital [16] (Table 7) and nongenital

Table 7. Reports of abnormalities of the human male genital system following intrauterine exposure to DES

| Kaplan [104] | 1959 | DES, 50—100 mg from 6 weeks to term and progesterone, 8—25 mg doses in early weeks of gestation | Single case report: full-term infant with hypospadias and undeveloped testes |
| Bibbo et al. [16] | 1977 | DES — dosage and timing of exposure variable | 41 of 163 exposed males had one or more: epididymal cysts, capsular induration, and/or hypotrophic testes, decreased sperm counts, and other abnormalities |

organs [84] when exposed to exogenous estrogens and progesterones. Unlike the effects on the female genitalia, in which the necessary exposure occurs during the first weeks of gestation, the abnormalities in the male, although not clearly dose-related, do not correspond with time of exposure [16].

Also a matter of concern is the possibility that the mothers who received DES may themselves be at exceptional risk of developing cancer[1].

The Prostate

Adenocarcinoma of the human prostate occurs almost exclusively in industrialized countries, where it is one of the most frequent causes of cancer deaths [210]. The epidemiologic features are similar to those of other hormone-dependent cancers (breast, endometrium, ovary) and those primary in the colon. Their incidence increases in immigrants and their offspring following migration from low- to high-incidence countries. In Japan, clinically significant prostate cancer is infrequent, but so-called latent cancer appears to be as frequent in Japan as in the United States [4]. These observations suggest that environmental carcinogens present in higher concentrations in Hawaii and the continental United States than in Japan increase the invasive character of cells that have already, through different influences, begun to proliferate and undergo other changes associated with invasive neoplasia. Another interpretation is that latent carcinoma is a separate entity not related to invasive cancer.

Cancer of the prostate is almost exclusively a disease of men older than 45 years; the United States death rates climb steeply after age 65. By age 85, the rates are twice those of men 10–15 years younger [28]. The age distribution and androgen-dependency of prostate cancer suggest that alterations in production or utilization of gonadotropic or gonadal hormones may be involved in the etiology, whatever the other "environmental" causes. Urinary androgens have been said to decrease in older men [148, 149], but other reports indicate that circulating testosterone does not decrease significantly in normal men even at advanced ages and the prostate maintains its ability to concentrate androgens from the plasma [135]. Prostate disorders are believed to begin with changes in uptake, retention, or utilization of androgens in the gland [135]. Cells of the normal human prostate, as do different androgen target organs, metabolize testosterone to 5α-dihydrotestosterone (DHT) and other metabolites. So far, no distinctive deletion or error in testosterone metabolism has been found to explain prostate cancer. DHT, which is even more active than testosterone, accumulates in the prostate of men past 60, particularly in the periurethral area [135].

How cancer is related to benign prostatic hypertrophy (BPH), a frequent disease, is unclear. While these two diseases share many epidemiologic features, e.g., their world distribution [210] and age of occurrence, they originate in different parts of the gland [148] — BPH in the periurethral area and carcinoma usually in the subcapsular portion that surrounds the periurethral component [148]. These components are believed to originate in different structures in the embryo and exhibit different patterns of hormone responsiveness. Some investigators have suggested that the periurethral area be considered the "female portion"

---

1 After the submission of this manuscript to the publisher, a report by BIBBO et al. (BIBBO, M., HAENSZEL, W. M., WIED, G. L., HUBBY, M., HERBST, A. L.: A twenty-five-year follow-up study of women exposed to diethylstilbestrol during pregnancy. New Engl. J. Med. *298*, 763–767 [1978]) indicated a slight, but statistically unsignificant, increase in breast cancers among women who took DES during pregnancy: 32 cancers in 693 exposed women and 21 in 668 unexposed.

(i.e., sensitive to estrogens and androgens), whereas the outer portion is the "true male prostate" (sensitive to androgens) [148]. The fetal prostate, in response to maternal hormones, undergoes reversible hypertrophy during the last trimester of pregnancy. The androgen-dependency of carcinoma, unlike BPH, can be readily demonstrated by the clinical response of at least some cancers to castration or treatment with estrogens. Both adenocarcinoma and BPH may be present in the same gland and occasionally carcinoma may originate in a hypertrophic nodule. Furthermore, carcinoma may invade the hypertrophied areas but does not ordinarily originate in cells of hypertrophic areas. BPH is not considered a precancerous lesion, although some relationship between BPH and cancer is suggested by one study of men with clinically significant BPH; subsequent death rates from prostate cancer were 3.7 times higher than men without the same degree of hypertrophy [8]. As mentioned earlier, concentrations of DHT are greater in hypertrophied than in normal glands [135], but I have found no reports that this is true in glands containing carcinoma.

In animals carcinoma of the prostate is rare, but it is occasionally observed in untreated dogs and rats [135]. The active androgen in the dog neoplasm is 5α-androstane-$3\alpha,17\alpha$-diol rather than 5α-dihydrotestosterone (DHT) as in man. Adenocarcinomas were observed in 7 of 41 aged rats (34—37 months) of the inbred A × C strain [185]. These carcinomas are not obvious on gross inspection and have not been observed to metastasize. Transplantable, metastasizing adenocarcinomas of the prostate have been observed in aged, random-bred, germ-free Lobund Wistar rats [170]. They have also been occasionally observed in untreated hamsters [185]. NOBLE [157, 158] produced a transplantable hormone-dependent adenocarcinoma of the prostate in rats of the inbred Nb strain by a combination of estrogens and androgens (estrone and testosterone propionate in cholesterol pellets implanted S.C.), although androgens alone will also induce them after a much longer latent period (17 months). A seventh generation transplant of the above-mentioned tumor is estrogen dependent rather than androgen dependent. Cancers of the prostate have been induced in rats by 20-methylcholanthrene and in hamsters, by SV40 virus. The latter are not considered acceptable models of the human neoplasm because of their inconsistent behavior and the lack of biologic and histopathologic identity with the human adenocarcinoma [135]. Prolactin and other pituitary and adrenocortical hormones known to affect the prostate may also play a role in carcinogenesis, but these areas have not been adequately studied.

The Testes

Neoplasms of the human testes are not known to be associated with preexisting abnormalities in production or utilization of hormones, although testicular neoplasms frequently *produce* gonadotropins or other hormones. The relatively high frequency of germ cell neoplasms in young men suggests a possible role of abnormal hormonal stimulation in their etiology, but there is no clear evidence to support this hypothesis. A possible relationship to an abnormal hormonal environment is suggested by relatively higher frequency of seminomas in cryptorchid testes [21]. Cryptorchidism is one result of exposure to DES in utero [16], but a positive history of such exposure accounts for only a small proportion of males with this abnormality. The men with genital system abnormalities resulting from fetal exposure to DES described in the report of BIBBO et al. [16] are very young and no excess of testicular or other neoplasm has been reported so far. Nevertheless, all men so exposed should be kept under close surveillance for many years because of this likely possibility. Pediatricians, urologists, and other physicians encountering cryptorchidism or testicular neoplasms should inquire about possible exposure to hormones. One unexplained feature of neoplasms of the human testes is their relative infrequency in American black men compared to white men [28].

Neoplasms of several types occur in the testes of animals. A high percent of rats of the F344 strain develop interstitial cell neoplasms [193], a type of neoplasm that is infrequent in the human. Interstitial cell neoplasms can also be induced in mice by S.C. implantation of DES pellets [187].

Neoplasms of other organs of the male genital system are infrequent in both men and animals and no evidence implicates abnormal hormonal stimulation in their etiology.

Other Hormone-target Organs

Neoplasms of the pituitary and thyroid glands are not known to be induced by hormones [61], although neoplasms originating in these organs frequently *produce* hormones. Transplantable adrenocortical tumors can be induced in rats by *estriol* [158, 159].

Nongenital Organs

Estrogens affect neoplasia in organs such as the liver [126], lymphoid tissue [63, 66, 113], skin [211], kidney [100], and urinary bladder [97]. Estrogen stimulation is suggested in some human nongenital neoplasms including those of salivary glands [42] and meninges [182] as evidenced by their greater frequency in women with breast cancer than previously expected. Receptors for growth hormone are present on human lymphocytes, probably T cells; the levels are increased in some children with acute lymphocytic leukemia [173].

Miscellaneous Sources of Exposure to Hormones and Hormonomimetic Compounds

In addition to endogenous hormones, humans and animals are also exposed to a variety of naturally occurring and synthetic compounds in foods, cosmetics, and drugs, characterized by an activity that, by various criteria, is similar to that of hormones. Table 8 lists some of these materials.

Phytoestrogens

SCHOENTAL [184] has listed plants (some commonly used as food for humans or animals) that contain compounds possessing estrogenic activity. Such compounds occur in date plam kernels, clovers, peanuts, carrots, soya beans, cereals, fruits, and other plants. Mycotoxins such as *zearalenone* (Fig. 10) produced by fungi that infect grains used for fodder can contaminate milk products or meat. Although none of these phytoestrogens are known to be carcinogenic [45], the wide distribution and opportunities for exposure to these plant products suggest that some of them might be involved in the induction of cancer. It would appear unlikely, however, that phytoestrogens cause cancer without some evidence of hyperestrogenism. So far, hyperestrogenism caused by phytoestrogens has been documented only in animals.

Table 8. Some compounds reported to display hormonal activity

Compound	Source	Reported activity
Phytoestrogens[a]:		
Estriol	Flowers of pussywillows (*Salix viminalis*), moghat roots, and date palm pollen grains [144]	
Estrone	Palm-kernel oil [97]	Uterine enlargement in mice [17, 18]
Coumarin derivatives[b]	Clovers and other plants [144]	Inhibition of reproduction of California quail [120]
Formononetin[b]	Leaves of stunted desert annuals [120], soybean meal (*Soja hispida*), and other plants [144]	"Clover disease" in sheep (dystocia, uterine prolapse, infertility, cystic changes in endometrium and cervix, galactorrhea) [1], inhibition of reproduction in California quail [120]
Genistein	Clovers, soya beans [184], and certain desert annuals [120]	
Zearalenone and related mycotoxins	Mycelia of the fungus *Gibberella zeae* (*Fusarium graminearum*), *Fusarium roseum*, and other *Fusaria* [80] that infect corn and other grains	Hyperestrogenism in swine (hyperplasia of uterus and mammary glands, vulvar tumefaction, squamous metaplasia of cervix and vagina) [154], infertility in cattle [146], reduction in egg production in hens [80], uterine enlargement in rats and mice [146]
Drugs:		
Digitalis preparations (powdered leaf, digitoxin, lanatoside C)	Leaves and seeds of *Digitalis purpurea* [144]	Gynecomastia [121], maturation of vaginal epithelium in postmenopausal women [111]
Methadone	Synthetic [144]	Gynecomastia [201]
Phenolphthalein, phenolphthalol	Synthetic [144]	Estrogenic activity as measured by the 18-h glycogen response in the rat uterus [20]

Drugs

An increased risk of breast cancer in women taking *Rauwolfia* alkaloids for hypertension has been claimed by some [9, 22, 83] and refuted by others [132, 163]. One author noted similarities in the structure of *reserpine* and those of known carcinogens [76]. Reserpine was

Compound	Source	Effects
Phenothiazines and other psychotropic drugs	Synthetic [144]	Human galactorrhea (male and female) [5, 15], amenorrhea [15], disturbances in lactation and estrus cycle in animals [15]
Rauwolfia derivatives	Root of *Rauwolfia serpentina* [144]	Possible increased risk of human breast cancer [9, 22, 83]
Spironolactone	Synthetic [144]	Gynecomastia, impotence in men [70, 130, 169], hirsutism [169], menstrual irregularities, breast soreness [130], and possibly increased risk of breast cancer [130] in women
Miscellaneous compounds:		
Aromatic polycyclic hydrocarbons (3,9-dihydrobenz[a]anthracene, 3,4-benzpyrene and others)	Mainly synthetic (coal tar derivatives) [6]	Induction of estrus in castrated mammals [6] and other techniques [181]
Chlorinated hydrocarbons (DDT analogs, polychlorinated biphenyls, and triphenyls)	Synthetic	18-h glycogen response in rat uterus [20]
Unidentified compounds	Dried flowering tops of *Cannabis sativa* [144]	Gynecomastia in young male heavy users of marijuana [78]

a Many other chemical compounds of plant origin exhibit activity that can, by various criteria, be considered estrogenic [23]. Laboratory techniques for assessing this activity are varied and not comparable between laboratories. The chemical structures vary widely and hormonal activity is not dependent on the steroid nucleus. See Fig. 10 for chemical formulas.

b This or related compounds used as drugs.

tested for carcinogenicity in mice of two strains [115]; when given orally, this drug was reported to accelerate development of mammary gland carcinomas in C3H mice but not in mice of a tumor-resistant strain designated XVIInc. Reserpine also accelerated the induction of hepatomas induced in rats by p-dimethylaminoazobenzene (DAB), whereas *iproniazid* retarded their development [114]. *Chlorpromazine* only slightly accelerated development of

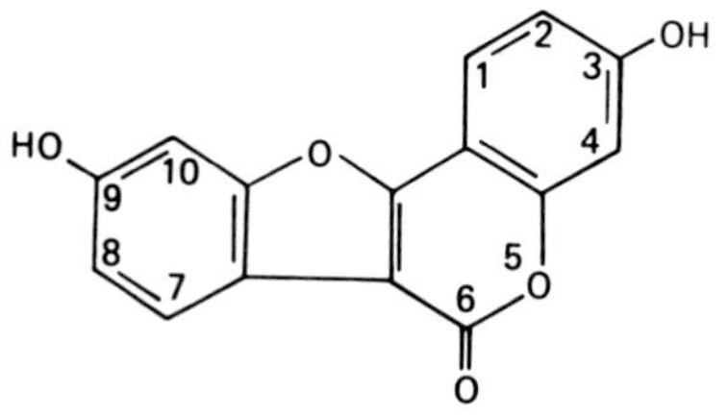

COUMESTROL 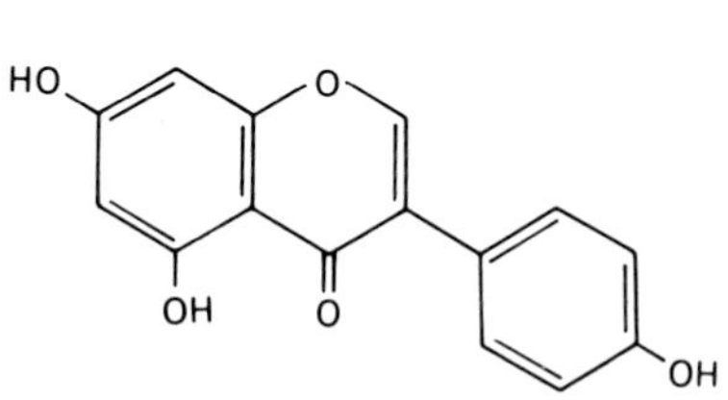   GENISTEIN

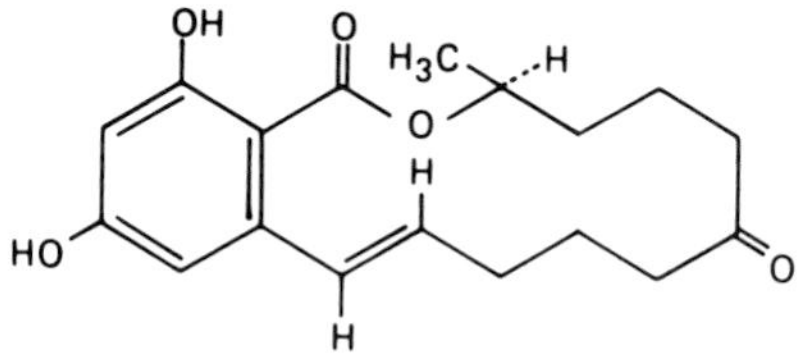

ZEARALENONE

Fig. 10. Compounds with estrogenic activity are found in a variety of plants

DAB-induced hepatomas in rats [116]. The WHO Information Bulletin #6 [209] lists three ongoing carcinogenicity studies of reserpine in rats, mice, and hamsters. Reserpine in daily doses of 5 or 10 µg/100 g resulted in decreased numbers and sizes of litters of rats and abnormalities in the vaginal smears, but did not affect lactation [67]. In other experiments reserpine (1 mg/kg S.C.), if given to rats at a critical point in time during proestrus, prevented ovulation by apparently blocking the release of pituitary gonadotropin [11].

Spironolactone, another antihypertensive drug, was linked to an increase in breast cancer in women in one study [130]. That this drug does have a stimulating effect on the mammary gland (perhaps indirectly) is illustrated by the fact that gynecomastia occurs in many male users of this drug [70]. The cause of the gynecomastia is uncertain, but one investigator suggested that it might be related to an alteration in drug-metabolizing oxidase P450 [124].

Gynecomastia has also been occasionally observed in men taking *digitalis* preparations [121] and in heavy users of marijuana [78].

Several psychotropic drugs induce abnormalities of the mammary glands and reproductive organs. *Galactorrhea* is sometimes a troublesome complication in men or women taking chlorpromazine, imipramine, and similar drugs singly or in combination [5]. Plasma prolactin levels were increased in 2 of 6 male patients with drug-associated galactorrhea in one study [5], and in 3 of 6 patients in another study [15]. Amenorrhea is another side effect sometimes noted in female patients taking these drugs. The mechanisms of these changes are not completely understood. Increased prolactin levels (higher in females than in males) have been detected in rats treated with psychotropic drugs. This increase may involve dopamine receptors since the release of prolactin from the adenohypophysis is normally inhibited by dopamine [32, 143]. CHU and SALMON [31] reported that cells in vaginal smears of hospitalized female mental patients contained a higher percent of cornified cells (evidence of estrogenicity) than did those of noninstitutionalized control women. This effect could not be

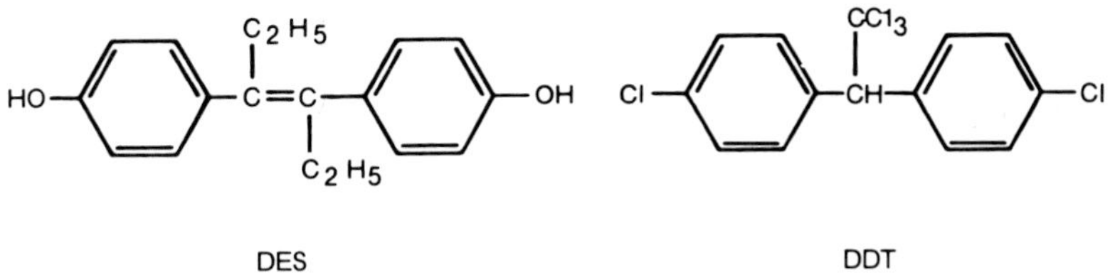

Fig. 11. Formulas for DES and DDT are similar

attributed to psychotropic drugs, but the mechanism is not known. Morphine is known to block ovulation and similar endogenous peptides in the brain (endorphins) that are involved in pain regulation stimulate the release of prolactin and growth hormone [69].

As shown in Table 8, a variety of synthetic chemical compounds display estrogenic activity including the insecticide DDT. Note the similarity of the formulas of DES and DDT (Fig. 11).

Conclusions

The mechanisms whereby estrogens and other hormones act as carcinogens or cocarcinogens are poorly understood. Although most evidence indicates that the carcinogenicity of DES is a manifestation of its estrogenicity, other stilbenes, such as 4-aminostilbene and 4-dimethylaminostilbene, are carcinogenic in several nongenital organs in rats [7]. ARCOS and ARGUS discuss the long-noted overlapping of estrogenicity and carcinogenicity of estrogens and polycyclic hydrocarbons [6].

Species, age, and sex differences affect the response of animals to hormones. For example, SHIMKIN and GRADY [186] noted that C57 black mice developed more extreme degrees of urinary retention, scrotal herniation, and pituitary adenomas in response to DES than did mice of strains A or C3H. Mice of strains A and C, but not C3H, develop primary testicular tumors (interstitial cell neoplasms) after exposure to estrogens [186]. DUNN and GREEN [44] noted the greater susceptibility of BALB/c strain mice to estrogen-induced carcinomas of the vagina-cervix than mice of other strains. The response of the mammary glands of mice to carcinogenic effects of hormones depends on contributing factors such as the presence of a virus and genetic characteristics.

One intriguing and as yet unexplained phenomenon is that most *human* neoplasms of nongenital organs are more frequent in *males* at all ages [98]. LILIENFELD [125] noted the greater frequencies in women of cancers of the thyroid and biliary system. He suggested that hormonal abnormalities may underlie the development of "masculine" cancers in women, i.e., those that are ordinarily more frequent in males, such as those of the larynx, lip, tongue, and lung. Such women, according to him, have a history of more abortions than women with "neutral" cancer, e.g., those of the colon, or "feminine" cancers, e.g., those of the thyroid or bile ducts. ASHLEY [10] advanced the interesting hypothesis that perhaps the female can better resist neoplasia because of immune factors located on X chromosomes. Because the female has two X chromosomes she has a better chance than the male to "recognize" and inactivate neoplastic cells in incipient stages. Other genes influencing susceptibility or resistance to cancer might also be located on sex chromosomes. In addition to genes coding for hormone synthesis and hormone receptors, the genes controlling production of enzymes that activate or inactivate chemical carcinogens may possibly also be located on sex chromosomes.

More information is needed to determine the precise roles of hormones and hormonomimetic compounds in carcinogenic processes in humans and animals. In the meantime, exposure to all of these should be reduced or eliminated wherever possible except for valid medical indications. All individuals receiving hormone medications should receive the lowest possible dose for the minimum time required to achieve the defined clinical objective and should remain under medical supervision while the medication is being taken and ideally for many years afterward under some type of surveillance, perhaps through the establishment of additional registries. To over-regulate the production and distribution of drugs composed of hormones makes no more sense than the outlawing of automobiles to prevent auto accidents, but rational decisions regarding the uses of these potent and frequently unpredictable compounds require more than a casual reappraisal of the purposes for which they are prescribed.

References

1. Adams, N. R.: Pathological changes in the tissues of infertile ewes with clover disease. J. Comp. Pathol. *86*, 29—35 (1976)
2. Adelman, R. C.: Impaired hormonal regulation of enzyme activity during aging. Fed. Proc. *34*, 179—182 (1975)
3. Adlercreutz, H., Tenhunen, R.: Some aspects of the interaction between natural and synthetic female sex hormones and the liver. Am. J. Med. *49*, 630—648 (1970)
4. Akazaki, K., Stemmermann, G. N.: Comparative study of latent carcinoma of the prostate among Japanese in Japan and Hawaii. J. Natl. Cancer Inst. *50*, 1137—1144 (1973)
5. Apostolakis, M., Kapetanakis, S., Lazos, G., Madena-Pyrgaki, A.: Plasma prolactin activity in male and female patients lactating due to psychotropic drug administration. Acta Endocrinol. Suppl. *155*, 19 (1971) (Abstract)
6. Arcos, J. C., Argus, M. F.: Chemical Induction of Cancer. Vol. IIA. New York and London: Academic Press, 1974a
7. Arcos, J. C., Argus, M. F.: Chemical Induction of Cancer. Vol. IIB. New York and London: Academic Press, 1974b
8. Armenian, H. K., Lilienfeld, A. M., Diamond, E. L., Bross, I. D. J.: Relation between benign prostatic hyperplasia and cancer of the prostate. Lancet *2*, 115—117 (1974)
9. Armstrong, B., Stevens, N., Doll, R.: Retrospective study of the association between use of rauwolfia derivatives and breast cancer in English women. Lancet *2*, 672—675 (1974)
10. Ashley, D. J. B.: A male-female differential in tumour incidence. Br. J. Cancer *23*, 21—25 (1969)
11. Barraclough, C. A.: Blockade of the release of pituitary gonadotropin by reserpine. Fed. Proc. *14*, 9—10 (1955)
12. Baum, J. K., Holtz, F., Bookstein, J. J., Klein, E. W.: Possible association between benign hepatomas and oral contraceptives. Lancet *2*, 926—929 (1973)
13. Beatson, G. T.: On the treatment of inoperable cases of carcinoma of the mamma: Suggestion for a new method of treatment with illustrative cases. Lancet *2*, 104—107 (1896)
14. Bern, H. A., Jones, L. A., Mills, K. T., Kohrman, A., Mori, T.: Use of the neonatal mouse in studying longterm effects of early exposure to hormones and other agents. J. Toxicol. Environ. Health Suppl. *1*, 103—116 (1976)
15. Beumont, P. J. V., Harris, G. W., Carr, P. J., Friesen, H. G., Kolakowska, T., Mackinnon, P. C. B., Mandelbrote, B. M., Wiles, D.: Some endocrine effects of phenothiazines; a preliminary report. J. Psychosom. Res. *16*, 297—304 (1972)

16. Bibbo, M., Gill, W. B., Azizi, F., Blough, R., Fang, V. S., Rosenfield, R. L., Schumacher, G. F. B., Sleeper, K., Sonek, M. G., Wied, G. L.: Follow-up study of male and female offspring of DES-exposed mothers. Obstet. Gynecol. *49*, 1–8 (1977)

17. Bickoff, E. M., Booth, A. N., Lyman, R. L., Livingston, A. L., Thompson, C. R., DeEds, F.: Coumestrol, a new estrogen isolated from forage crops. Science *126*, 969–970 (1957)

18. Bickoff, E. M., Livingston, A. L., Hendrickson, A. P., Booth, A. N.: Relative potencies of several estrogenlike compounds found in forages. J. Agric. Food Chem. *10*, 410–412 (1962)

19. Bird, D. R., Vowles, K. D. J.: Liver damage from long term methyltestosterone. Lancet *2*, 400–401 (1977)

20. Bitman, J., Cecil, H. C.: Estrogenic activity of DDT analogs and polychlorinated biphenyls. J. Agric. Food Chem. *18*, 1108–1112 (1970)

21. Bolande, R. P.: Childhood tumors and their relationship to birth defects. In Genetics of Human Cancer. Mulvihill, J. J., Miller, R. W., Fraumeni, J. F., Jr. (Eds.). New York: Raven Press, 1977

22. Boston Collaborative Drug Program. Reserpine and breast cancer. Lancet *2*, 669–671 (1974)

23. Bradbury, R. B., White, D. E.: Estrogens and related substances in plants. Vitam. Horm. *12*, 207–233 (1954)

24. Brooks, S. C.: The metabolism of steroid hormones in breast cancer: A reappraisal. Curr. Top. Mol. Endocrinol. *4*, 36–50 (1976)

25. Budzynska, A., Wasikowa, R., Zajac, J.: Hyperestrogenism in children of employees of the Polfa Pharmaceutical Laboratories in Jenenia Gora. Pol. Med. J. *6*, 1249–1256 (1967)

26. Buell, P.: Changing incidence of breast cancer in Japanese-American women. J. Natl. Cancer Inst. *51*, 1479–1483 (1973)

27. Buell, P., Dunn, J. E.: Cancer mortality among Japanese issei and nisei of California. Cancer *18*, 656–664 (1965)

28. Burbank, F.: Patterns in Cancer Mortality in the United States: 1950–1967. Natl. Cancer Inst. Monogr. *33*, 307 (1971)

29. Carcinogenicity Testing of Oral Contraceptives. Report by the Committee on Safety of Medicines. London: Her Majesty's Stationery Office, 1972

30. Chen, H. J., Bradley, C. J., Meites, J.: Stimulation of growth of carcinogen-induced mammary cancers in rats by thyrotropin-releasing hormone. Cancer Res. *37*, 64–66 (1977)

31. Chu, E. W., Salmon, M. J.: Observations on vaginal cornification in patients resident in a mental hospital. Am. J. Obstet. Gynecol. *83*, 165–170 (1962)

32. Clemens, J. A., Smalstig, E. B., Sawyer, B. D.: Antipsychotic drugs stimulate prolactin release. Psychopharmacologia (Berl.) *40*, 123–127 (1974)

33. Conney, A. H., Burns, J. J.: Metabolic interactions among environmental chemicals and drugs. Science *178*, 576–586 (1972)

34. Corbett, D. G., Abrams, E. W.: Bilateral carcinoma of the male breast associated with prolonged stilbestrol therapy for carcinoma of the prostate. J. Urol. *64*, 377–381 (1950)

35. Costlow, M. E., McGuire, W. L.: Autoradiographic localization of prolactin receptors in 7,12-dimethylbenz[a]anthracene-induced rat mammary carcinoma. J. Natl. Cancer Inst. *58*, 1173–1175 (1977)

36. Cutler, B. S., Forbes, A. P., Ingersoll, F. M., Scully, R. E.: Endometrial carcinoma after stilbestrol therapy in gonadal dysgenesis. New Engl. J. Med. *287*, 628–631 (1972)

37. Dao, T. L., Morreal, C., Nemoto, T.: Urinary estrogen excretion in men with breast cancer. New Engl. J. Med. *289*, 138–140 (1973)

38. Dean, L., Abell, D. A., Beischer, N. A.: Incidence of anencephaly and other major malformations when oestriol excretion is very low. Br. Med. J. *1*, 257–258 (1977)

39. Diczfalusy, E.: Recent progress in the fetoplacental metabolism of steroids. In: Reproductive Endocrinology. Vokaer, R., DeBock, G. (Eds.). New York: Pergamon Press, 1975, p. 3

40. Dodds, E. C., Golberg, L., Lawson, W., Robinson, R.: Oestrogenic activity of certain synthetic compounds. Nature (London) *141*, 247–248 (1938)

41. Doisy, E. A., Veler, C. D., Thayer, S.: Folliculin from urine of pregnant women. Am. J. Physiol. *90*, 329–330 (1929)

42. Dunn, J. E., Jr., Bragg, K. U., Sautter, C., Gardipee, C.: Breast cancer risk following a major salivary gland carcinoma. Cancer *29*, 1343–1346 (1972)

43. Dunn, T. B.: Cancer of the uterine cervix in mice fed a liquid diet containing an antifertility drug. J. Natl. Cancer Inst. *43*, 671–692 (1969)

44. Dunn, T. B., Green, A. W.: Cysts of the epididymis, cancer of the cervix, granular cell myoblastoma, and other lesions after estrogen injection in newborn mice. J. Natl. Cancer Inst. *31*, 425–455 (1963)

45. Edgren, R. A.: Are oral contraceptives and diethylstilbestrol (DES) involved in sex-linked cancer? Curr. Top. Mol. Endocrinol. *4*, 95–106 (1976)

46. Editorial: Cyproterone acetate. Lancet *1*, 1003–1004 (1976)

47. Edmondson, H. A.: Tumors of the Gallbladder and Extrahepatic Bile Ducts. In: Atlas of Tumor Pathology, Section VII, Fascicle 26. Washington, D.C.: Armed Forces Inst. Pathol., 1967

48. Eidelsberg, J.: Estrogens in urine and cytology of vaginal smears after the use of an estrogenic cream. Am. J. Med. Sci. *214*, 630–632 (1947)

49. Eisenfeld, A. J., Aten, R., Weinberger, M., Haselbacher, G., Halpern, K., Krakoff, L.: Estrogen receptor in the mammalian liver. Science *191*, 862–865 (1976)

50. Everson, R. B., Li, F. P., Fraumeni, J. F., Jr., Fishman, J., Wilson, R. E., Stout, D., Norris, H. J.: Familial male breast cancer. Lancet *1*, 9–12 (1976)

51. Faber, L. E., Saffran, J., Chen, T. J., Leavitt, W. W.: Mammalian progesterone receptors: Biosynthesis, structure and nuclear binding. Curr. Top. Mol. Endocrinol. *4*, 68–84 (1976)

52. Farrell, G. C., Joshua, D. E., Uren, R. F., Baird, P. J., Perkins, K. W., Kronerberg, H.: Androgen-induced hepatoma. Lancet *1*, 430–432 (1975)

53. Fechner, R. E.: Carcinoma of the breast during estrogen replacement therapy. Cancer *29*, 566–573 (1972)

54. Fechner, R. E.: Influence of oral contraceptives on breast diseases. Cancer *39*, 2764–2771 (1977)

55. Festing, M., Staats, J.: Standardized nomenclature for inbred strains of rats. Transplantation *16*, 221–245 (1973)

56. Fitzsimons, M. P.: Gynaecomastia in stilboestrol workers. Br. J. Ind. Med. *1*, 235–237 (1945)

57. Forsberg, J.-G.: Derivation and differentiation of the vaginal epithelium. Lund, The Institute of Anatomy (Thesis), 1963

58. Forsberg, J.-G.: Induction of conditions leading to cancer in the genital tract by estrogen during the differentiation phase of the genital epithelium. Adv. Biosci. *13*, 139–151 (1974)

59. Forsberg, J.-G.: Animal model: Estrogen-induced adenosis of vagina and cervix in mice. Am. J. Pathol. *84*, 669–672 (1976)

60. Fotherby, K.: Metabolism of synthetic steroids by animals and man. Acta Endocrinol. Suppl. *185*, 119–147 (1974)

61. Foulds, L.: Neoplastic Development, Vol. 2. New York: Academic Press, 1975

62. Fraumeni, J. F., Lloyd, J. W., Smith, E. M., Wagoner, J. K.: Cancer mortality among nuns: Role of marital status in etiology of neoplastic disease in women. J. Natl. Cancer Inst. *42*, 455–468 (1969)

63. Furth, J.: Recent experimental studies on leukosis. Physiol. Rev. *26*, 47–76 (1946)

64. Gardner, W. U., Allen, E.: Malignant and non-malignant uterine and vaginal lesions in mice receiving estrogens and estrogens and androgens simultaneously. Yale J. Biol. Med. *12*, 213–234 (1939)

65. Gardner, W. U., Pan, S. C.: Malignant tumors of the uterus and vagina in untreated mice of the PM stock. Cancer Res. *8*, 241–256 (1948)

66. Gardner, W. U., Dougherty, T. F., Williams, W. L.: Lymphoid tumors in mice receiving steroid hormones. Cancer Res. *4*, 73—87 (1944)
67. Gaunt, R., Renzi, A. A., Antonchak, N., Miller, G. J., Gilman, M.: Endocrine aspects of the pharmacology of reserpine. Ann. N.Y. Acad. Sci. *59*, 22—35 (1954)
68. Gillette, J. R., Stripp, B.: Pre- and postnatal enzyme capacity for drug metabolite production. Fed. Proc. *34*, 172—178 (1975)
69. Grandison, L., Guidotti, A.: Regulation of prolactin release by endogenous opiates. Nature (London) *270*, 357—359 (1977)
70. Greenblatt, D. J., Koch-Weser, J.: Adverse reactions to spironolactone. A report from the Boston Collaborative Drug Surveillance Program. J. Am. Med. Assoc. *225*, 40—43 (1973)
71. Greenblatt, R. B., Brown, N. H.: The storage of estrogen in human fat after estrogen administration. Am. J. Obstet. Gynecol. *63*, 1361—1363 (1952)
72. Greene, H. S. N.: Diseases of the rabbit. In: Pathology of Laboratory Animals. Ribelin, W. E., McCoy, J. R. (Eds.). Springfield: Charles C. Thomas, 1965, p. 330
73. Grumbach, M. M.: Gonads. Sex determination and sex differentiation. In: Textbook of Medicine. Beeson, P.B., McDermott, W. (Eds.). Philadelphia and London: W. B. Saunders Co., 1963, p. 1407
74. Gupta, R. L.: Carcinoma of the breast in a case of Klinefelter syndrome. Indian J. Cancer *3*, 184—189 (1966)
75. Gustafsson, J., Stenberg, A.: Partial masculinization of rat liver enzyme activities following treatment with FSH. Endocrinology *96*, 501—504 (1975)
76. Hadler, H. I.: Reserpine and chemical carcinogenesis. Lancet *1*, 169 (1975)
77. Haenszel, W., Kurihara, M.: Studies of Japanese migrants. I. Mortality from cancer and other diseases among Japanese in the United States. J. Natl. Cancer Inst. *40*, 43—68 (1968)
78. Harmon, J., Aliapoulios, M. A.: Gynecomastia in marijuana users. New Engl. J. Med. *287*, 936 (1972)
79. Harry, R. G.: Modern Cosmetology, Vol. 1. New York: Chemical Publishing Co., 1968
80. Harwig, J., Munro, I. C.: Mycotoxins of possible importance in diseases of Canadian farm animals. Can. Vet. J. *16*, 125—139 (1975)
81. Hausknecht, R. U., Gusberg, S. B.: Estrogen metabolism in patients at high risk for endometrial carcinoma. Am. J. Obstet. Gynecol. *116*, 981—984 (1973)
82. Heath, E. C., Dingell, J. V.: The interaction of foreign chemical compounds with the glucuronidation of estrogens in vitro. Drug Metab. Dispos. *2*, 556—565 (1974)
83. Heinonen, O. P., Shapiro, S., Tuonimen, L., Turunen, M. I.: Reserpine use in relation to breast cancer. Lancet *2*, 675—677 (1974)
84. Heinonen, O. P., Slone, D., Monson, R. R., Hook, E. B., Shapiro, S.: Cardiovascular birth defects and antenatal exposure to female sex hormones. New Engl. J. Med. *296*, 67—70 (1977)
85. Helton, E. D., Goldzieher, J. W.: The pharmacokinetics of ethynyl estrogens. A review. Contraception *15*, 255—284 (1977)
86. Henderson, B. E., Gerkins, V. R., Pike, M. C.: Sexual factors and pregnancy. In: Persons at High Risk of Cancer. Fraumeni, J. F. (Ed.). New York: Academic Press, Inc., 1975, p. 267
87. Herbst, A. L., Ulfelder, H., Poskanzer, D. C.: Adenocarcinoma of the vagina. Association of maternal stilbestrol therapy with tumor appearance in young women. New Engl. J. Med. *284*, 878—881 (1971)
88. Hertig, A. T., Gore, H.: Tumors of the female sex organs. Part 2. Tumors of the vulva, vagina and uterus. In: Atlas of Tumor Pathology, Section IX, Fascicle 33. Washington, D.C.: Armed Forces Inst. of Pathol., 1960
89. Hertz, R.: Steroid-induced, steroid-producing, and steroid-responsive tumors. Curr. Top. Mol. Endocrinol. *4*, 1—14 (1976)
90. Heston, W. E., Vlahakis, G., Desmukes, B.: Effects of the antifertility drug Enovid in five strains of mice, with particular regard to carcinogenesis. J. Natl. Cancer Inst. *51*, 209—224 (1973)

91.. Hill, M. J., Goddard, P., Williams, R. E. O.: Gut bacteria and etiology of cancer of the breast. Lancet 2, 472—473 (1971)

92. Hoover, R., Fraumeni, J. F., Jr., Everson, R., Myers, M. H.: Cancer of the uterine corpus after hormonal treatment for breast cancer. Lancet 1, 885—887 (1976)

93. Hoover, R., Gray, L. A., Cole, P., MacMahon, B.: Menopausal estrogens and breast cancer. New Engl. J. Med. 295, 401—405 (1976)

94. Hoover, R., Gray, L. A., Sr., Fraumeni, J. F.: Stilboestrol (diethylstilboestrol) and the risk of ovarian cancer. Lancet 2, 533—534 (1977)

95. Huseby, R. A.: Estrogen-induced Leydig cell tumor in the mouse: A model system for the study of carcinogenesis and hormone dependency. J. Toxicol. Environ. Health, Suppl. 1, 177—192 (1976)

96. Ingelfinger, F. J.: Gallstones and estrogens. New Engl. J. Med. 290, 51—52 (1974)

97. International Agency for Research on Cancer. IARC Monographs on the Evaluation of Carcinogenic Risk of Chemicals to Man. Sex Hormones, Vol. 6. Lyon: International Agency for Research on Cancer, 1974

98. International Agency for Research on Cancer, World Health Organization. Cancer Incidence in Five Continents, Vol. III. Waterhouse, J., Muir, C., Correa, P., Powell, J. (Eds.). IARC Scientific Publications No. 15. Lyon: International Agency for Research on Cancer, 1976

99. Jackson, A. W., Muldal, S., Ockey, C. H., O'Connor, P. J.: Carcinoma of male breast in association with the Klinefelter syndrome. Br. Med. J. 1, 223—225 (1965)

100. Jasmin, G., Riopelle, J. L.: Nephroblastomas induced in ovariectomized rats by dimethylbenzanthracene. Cancer Res. 30, 321—326 (1970)

101. Joly, D., Lilienfeld, A. J., Diamond, E. L., Bross, I. D.: An epidemiologic study of the relationship of reproductive experience with cancer of the ovary. Am. J. Epidemiol. 99, 190—209 (1974)

102. Jones, L. A., Bern, H. A.: Long-term effects of neonatal treatment with progesterone, alone and in combination with estrogen, on the mammary gland and reproductive tract of female BALB/cfC3H mice. Cancer Res. 37, 67—75 (1977)

103. Jørgensen, P. I.: Low urinary oestriol excretion during pregnancy in women giving birth to infants with Down's syndrome. Lancet 2, 782—783 (1972)

104. Kaplan, N. M.: Male pseudohermaphrodism. Report of a case with observations on pathogenesis. New Engl. J. Med. 261, 641—644 (1959)

105. Kimura, T., Nandi, S.: Nature of induced persistent vaginal cornification in mice. IV. Changes in the vaginal epithelium of old mice treated neonatally with estradiol or testosterone. J. Natl. Cancer Inst. 39, 75—93 (1967)

106. King, N. W.: Comparative pathology of the uterus. In: The Uterus. Norris, H. J., Hertig, A. T., Abel, M. R. (Eds.). Baltimore: Williams and Wilkins, 1973, p. 489

107. Kirschner, M. A.: The role of hormones in the etiology of human breast cancer. Cancer 39, 2716—2726 (1977)

108. Kling, R. E., Lazar, A.: The development of a radioimmunometric assay for diethylstilbestrol in tissues: Part I. FDA By-Lines, No. 2, September 1976, p. 65

109. Kodama, M., Kodama, T., Totani, R.: Hormonal status of cervical cancer. J. Natl. Cancer Inst. 59, 41—47 (1977)

110. Koo, G. C., Wachtel, S. S., Saenger, P., New, M. I., Dosik, H., Amarose, A. P., Dorus, E., Ventruto, V.: H—Y Antigen: Expression in human subjects with the testicular feminization syndrome. Science 196, 655—656 (1977)

111. Koss, L. G.: Diagnostic Cytology and its Histopathologic Bases. Philadelphia: Lippincott, 1968

112. Kupfer, D., Bulger, W. H.: Interactions of chlorinated hydrocarbons with steroid hormones. Fed. Proc. 35, 2603—2608 (1976)

113. Lacassagne, A.: Sarcomes lymphoides apparus chez des souris longuement traitées par des hormones oestrogenes. C.R. Soc. Biol. Paris 126, 193—195 (1937)

114. Lacassagne, A.: Effets opposés de l'iproniazide et de la resérpine, sur la cancérisation du foie du rat par p-dimethylaminoazobenzene. C.R. Acad. Sci. Paris *263*, 701—703 (series D) (1966)

115. Lacassagne, A., Duplan, J.-F.: Le mécanisme de la cancérisation de la mamelle chez la souris, considéré d'apres les résultats d'experiences au moyen de la reserpine. Compt. Rend. *249*, 810—812 (1959)

116. Lacassagne, A., Hurst, L., Rosenberg, A.-J.: Influence de la chlorpromazine et de la reserpine sur la cancerisation experimentale du foie chez le rat. Compt. Rend. *249*, 903—905 (1959)

117. Lacassagne, M. A.: Apparition de cancers de la mamelle chez la souris mâle, soumise à des injections de folliculine. Compt. Rend. Acad. Sci. *195*, 630—632 (1932)

118. Lathrop, A. E. C., Loeb, L.: Further investigations on the origin of tumors in mice. III. On the part played by internal secretion in the spontaneous development of tumors. J. Cancer Res. *1*, 1—19 (1916)

119. Leonard, B. J.: The use of rodents for studies of toxicity in contraceptive research. Acta Endocrinol. Suppl. *185*, 34—73 (1974)

120. Leopold, A. S., Erwin, M., Oh, J., Browning, B.: Phytoestrogens: Adverse effects on reproduction in California quail. Science *191*, 98—100 (1976)

121. LeWinn, E. B.: Gynecomastia during digitalis therapy. New Engl. J. Med. *248*, 316—320 (1953)

122. Lewis, R. M.: The clinical use of stilbestrol, a synthetic estrogen. Preliminary report. Yale J. Biol. Med. *12*, 235—238 (1939)

123. Liao, S., Hung, S. C., Tymoczko, J. L., Liang, T.: Active forms and biodynamics of the androgen-receptor in various target tissues. Curr. Top. Mol. Endocrinol. *4*, 139—151 (1976)

124. Licata, A. A., Bartter, F. C.: Spironolactone-induced gynaecomastia related to allergic reaction to 'Darvon compound'. Lancet *2*, 905 (1976)

125. Lilienfeld, A. M.: Possible existence or predisposing factors in the etiology of selected cancers of non-sexual sites in females: A preliminary inquiry. Cancer *9*, 111—122 (1956)

126. Lingeman, C. H.: Liver-cell neoplasms and oral contraceptives. Lancet *1*, 64 (1974a)

127. Lingeman, C. H.: Etiology of cancer of the ovary: A review. J. Natl. Cancer Inst. *53*, 1603—1618 (1974b)

128. Lippman, M., Barr, R.: Glucocorticoid receptors in purified subpopulations of human peripheral blood lymphocytes. J. Immunol. *118*, 1977—1981 (1977)

129. Lippman, M. E., Osborne, C. K., Knazek, R., Young, N.: In vitro model systems for the study at hormone-dependent human breast cancer. New Engl. J. Med. *296*, 154—159 (1977)

130. Loube, S. D., Quirk, R. A.: Breast cancer associated with administration of spironolactone. Lancet *1*, 1428—1429 (1975)

131. Lyon, F. A.: Development of adenocarcinoma of endometrium in young women receiving long-term sequential oral contraception. Am. J. Obstet. Gynecol. *123*, 299—301 (1975)

132. Mack, T. M., Henderson, B. E., Gerkins, V. R., Arthur, M., Baptista, J., Pike, M. C.: Reserpine and breast cancer in a retirement community. New Engl. J. Med. *292*, 1366—1371 (1975)

133. MacMahon, B., Austin, J. H.: Association of carcinomas of breast and corpus uteri. Cancer *23*, 275—280 (1969)

134. MacMahon, B., Cole, P., Brown, J.: Etiology of human breast cancer: A review. J. Natl. Cancer Inst. *50*, 21—42 (1973)

135. Mainwaring, W. I. P.: The relevance of studies on androgen action to prostatic cancer. Curr. Top. Mol. Endocrinol. *4*, 152—171 (1976)

136. McCarty, K. S., Jr., McCarty, K. S.: Steroid hormone receptors in the regulation of differentiation. A review. Am. J. Pathol. *86*, 703—744 (1977)

137. McGuire, W. L., Horwitz, K. B., Pearson, O. H., Segaloff, A.: Current status of estrogen and progesterone receptors in breast cancer. Cancer *39*, 2934—2947 (1977)

138. McKinney, G. R., Weikel, J. H., Webb, W. K., Dick, R. G.: Use of life-table techniques to estimate effects of certain steroids on probability of tumor formation in a long term study in rats. Toxicol. Appl. Pharmacol. *12*, 68—79 (1968)

139. McLachlan, J. A.: Transplacental toxicity of diethylstilbestrol: A special problem in safety evaluation. Adv. Modern Toxicol. *1*, 423–448 (1976)

140. McLachlan, J. A., Newbold, R. R., Bullock, B.: Reproductive tract lesions in male mice exposed prenatally to diethylstilbestrol. Science *190*, 991–992 (1975)

141. McLean, A. E. M.: Enzyme induction in the fetus and the role of enzyme induction in the localization of carcinogenesis. In: Transplacental Carcinogenesis. Tomatis, L., Mohr, U. (Eds.). Lyon: International Agency for Research on Cancer, 1973

142. Meissner, W. A., Sommers, S. C., Sherman, G.: Endometrial hyperplasia, endometrial carcinoma and endometriosis produced experimentally by estrogen. Cancer *10*, 500–509 (1957)

143. Meltzer, H. Y., Sachar, E. J., Frantz, A. G.: Dopamine antagonism by thioridazine in schizophrenia. Biol. Psychiatry *10*, 53–57 (1975)

144. The Merck Index, 9th Ed., Windholz, M. (Ed.). Rahway: Merck and Co., 1976

145. Migaki, G., Carey, A. M., Turnquest, R. U., Garner, F. M.: Pathology of bovine uterine adenocarcinoma. J. Am. Vet. Med. Assoc. *157*, 1577–1584 (1970)

146. Mirocha, C. J., Christensen, C. M., Nelson, G. H.: Physiologic activity of some fungal estrogens produced by Fusarium. Cancer Res. *28*, 2319–2322 (1968)

147. Moore, C. R., Lamar, J. K., Beck, N.: Cutaneous absorption of sex hormones. J. Am. Med. Assoc. *111*, 11–14 (1938)

148. Mostofi, F. K., Leestma, J. E.: Lower urinary tract and male genitalia. In: Pathology, sixth edition, Vol. 1. Anderson, W. A. D. (Ed.). St. Louis: C.V. Mosby, 1971, p. 828

149. Mostofi, F. K., Price, E. B: Tumors of the male genital system. In: Atlas of Tumor Pathology, second series, Fascicle 8. Washington, D.C.: Armed Forces Inst. Pathol., 1973

150. Mulvihill, J. J.: Congenital and genetic diseases. In: Persons at High Risk of Cancer. Fraumeni, J. F. (Ed.). New York: Academic Press, 1975, p. 3

151. Murphy, E. D.: Carcinogenesis of the uterine cervix in mice. Effect of diethylstilbesterol after limited application of 3-methylcholanthrene. J. Natl. Cancer Inst. *27*, 611–653 (1961)

152. Murphy, E. D.: Carcinogenesis of the uterine cervix in mice: Effect of castration after limited application of 3-methylcholanthrene. J. Natl. Cancer Inst. *41*, 1111–1116 (1968)

153. Nadell, J., Kosek, J.: Peliosis hepatis. Twelve cases associated with oral androgen therapy. Arch. Pathol. Lab. Med. *101*, 405–410 (1977)

154. Nelson, G. H., Christensen, C. M., Mirocha, C.: Fusarium and estrogenism in swine. J. Am. Vet. Med. Assoc. *163*, 1276–1277 (1973)

155. Neumann, F., Gräf, K. J.: Discovery, development, mode of action and clinical uses of cyproterone acetate. J. Int. Med. Res. *3* (Suppl. 4), 1–9 (1975)

156. Nicolis, G. L., Sabetghadam, R., Hsu, C. C. S., Sohval, A. R., Gabrilove, J. L.: Breast cancer after mumps orchitis. J. Am. Med. Assoc. *223*, 1032–1033 (1973)

157. Noble, R. L.: The development of prostatic adenocarcinoma in Nb rats following prolonged sex hormone administration. Cancer Res. *37*, 1929–1933 (1957)

158. Noble, R. L.: A new approach to the hormonal cause and control of experimental carcinomas, including those of the breast. Ann. R. Coll. Phys. Surg. Can. *9*, 169–180 (1976)

159. Noble, R. L.: Hormonal control of growth and progression in tumors of Nb rats and a theory of action. Cancer Res. *37*, 82–94 (1977)

160. Nomura, T., Kanzaki, T.: Induction of urogenital anomalies and some tumors in the progeny of mice receiving diethylstilbestrol during pregnancy. Cancer Res. *37*, 1099–1104 (1977)

161. Nomura, Y., Kobayashi, S., Takatani, O., Sugano, H., Matsumoto, K., McGuire, W. L.: Estrogen receptor and endocrine responsiveness in Japanese versus American breast cancer patients. Cancer Res. *37*, 106–110 (1977)

162. Norris, H. J., Taylor, H. B.: Carcinoma of the male breast. Cancer *23*, 1428–1435 (1969)

163. O'Fallon, W. M., Labarthe, D. R., Kurland, L. T.: Rauwolfia derivatives and breast cancer. Lancet *2*, 292–300 (1975)

164. O'Shea, J. D., Jabara, A. G.: The histogenesis of canine ovarian tumours induced by stilboestrol administration. Pathol. Vet. *4*, 137–148 (1967)

165. Otten, J., Smets, R., Jager, R. de, Gerard, A., Maurus, R.: Hepatoblastoma in an infant after contraceptive intake during pregnancy. New Engl. J. Med. *297*, 222 (1977)

166. Overholser, M. D., Allen, E.: Atypical growth induced in cervical epithelium of the monkey by prolonged injection of ovarian hormone combined with chronic trauma. Surg. Gynecol. Obstet. *60*, 129—136 (1935)

167. Persijn, R. P., Korsten, C. B., Engelsman, E.: Oestrogen and androgen receptors in breast cancer. Br. Med. J. *4*, 503 (1975)

168. Petit, P., Engels, J.: Low maternal oestriol excretion and congenital chromosome abnormalities. Lancet *2*, 970 (1972)

169. Physicians Desk Reference, 31st Edition. Oradell, N. J., Medical Economics Co., 1977

170. Pollard, M., Luckert, P. H.: Transplantable metastasizing prostate adenocarcinomas in rats. J. Natl. Cancer Inst. *54*, 643—649 (1975)

171. Poortman, J., Prenan, J. A. C., Schwarz, F., Thijssen, J. H. H.: Interaction of $\triangle^5$-androstene-3β, 17β-diol with estradiol and dihydrotestosterone receptors in human myometrial and mammary cancer tissue. J. Clin. Endocrinol. Metab. *40*, 373—379 (1975)

172. Pryor, A. C., Cohen, R. J., Goldman, R. L.: Hepatocellular carcinoma in a woman on long term oral contraceptives. Cancer *40*, 884—888 (1977)

173. Rogers, P. C., Komp, D., Rogol, A., Sabio, H.: Possible effects of growth hormone on development of acute lymphoblastic leukaemia. Lancet *2*, 434—435 (1977)

174. Rudali, G., Apiou, F., Muel, B.: Mammary cancer produced in mice with estriol. Eur. J. Cancer *11*, 39—41 (1975)

175. Russfield, A. B.: Tumors of Endocrine Glands and Secondary Sex Organs. Washington, D.C.: USPHS, Department HEW, 1966

176. Rustia, M., Shubik, P.: Transplacental effects of diethylstilbestrol on the genital tract of hamster offspring. Cancer Lett. *1*, 139—146 (1976)

177. Schaffer, A. J., Avery, M. E.: Diseases of the Newborn. Third Edition. Philadelphia: Saunders, 1971

178. Schardein, J. L., Kaump, D. H., Woosley, E. T., Jellema, M. M.: Long-term toxicologic and tumorigenesis studies on an oral contraceptive agent in albino rats. Toxicol. Appl. Pharmacol. *16*, 10—23 (1970)

179. Scheike, O.: Male breast cancer. Acta Pathol. Microbiol. Scand., Section A, Suppl. *251*, 13—35 (1975)

180. Schindler, A. E.: Steroid metabolism of fetal tissues. II. Conversion of androstenedione to estrone. Am. J. Obstet. Gynecol. *123*, 265—268 (1975)

181. Schneider, S. L., Alks, V., Morreal, C. E., Sinha, D. K., Dao, T. L.: Estrogenic properties of 3,9-dihydroxybenz[a]anthracene, a potential metabolite of benz[a]anthracene. J. Natl. Cancer Inst. *57*, 1351—1354 (1976)

182. Schoenberg, B. S., Christine, B. W., Whisnant, J. P.: Nervous system neoplasms and primary malignancies of other sites. Neurology *25*, 705—712 (1975)

183. Schoenberg, B. S., Greenberg, R. A., Eisenberg, H.: Occurrence of certain multiple primary cancers in females. J. Natl. Cancer Inst. *43*, 5—32 (1969)

184. Schoental, R.: Carcinogenic hazards of estrogens. In: Multiple Primary Malignant Tumours. Severi, L. (Ed.). Perugia: Division of Cancer Research, 1974, p. 1003

185. Shain, S. A., McCullough, B., Segaloff, A.: Spontaneous adenocarcinoma of the ventral prostate of aged A X C rats. J. Natl. Cancer Inst. *55*, 177—180 (1975)

186. Shimkin, M. B., Grady, H. G.: Toxic and carcinogen effects of stilbestrol in strain C3H male mice. J. Natl. Cancer Inst. *2*, 55—60 (1941)

187. Shimkin, M. B., Grady, H. G., Andervont, H. B.: Induction of testicular tumors and other effects of stilbestrol-cholesterol pellets in strain C mice. J. Natl. Cancer Inst. *2*, 65—80 (1941)

188. Silverberg, S. G., Makowski, E. L.: Endometrial carcinoma in young women taking oral contraceptive agents. Obstet. Gynecol. *46*, 503—506 (1975)

189. Smith, D. C., Prentice, R., Thompson, D. J., Herrmann, W. L.: Association of exogenous estrogen and endometrial carcinoma. New Engl. J. Med. *293*, 1164—1167 (1975)

190. Smith, O. W., Smith, G. V. S., Hurwitz, D.: Increased excretion of pregnanediol in pregnancy from diethylstilbestrol with special reference to the prevention of late pregnancy accidents. Am. J. Obstet. Gynecol. *51*, 411—415 (1946)

191. Smith, R. L.: Biliary excretion and hepatotoxicity of contraceptive steroids. Acta Endocrinol. Suppl. *185*, 149—168 (1974)

192. Smithline, F., Sherman, L., Kolodny, H. D.: Prolactin and breast carcinoma. New Engl. J. Med. *292*, 784—792 (1975)

193. Snell, K. C.: Spontaneous lesion of the rat. In: Pathology of Laboratory Animals. Ribelin, W. E., McCoy, J. R. (Eds.). Springfield: Charles C. Thomas, 1965, p. 266

194. Song, C. S., Kappas, A.: The influence of hormones on hepatic function. In: Progress in Liver Diseases, 1971, Vol. 3, p. 89

195. Stangel, J. J., Innerfield, I., Reyniak, J. U., Stone, M. L.: The effect of conjugated estrogens on coagulability in menopausal women. Obstet. Gynecol. *49*, 314—316 (1977)

196. Stumpf, W. E., Sar, M., Aumüller, G.: The heart: A target organ for estradiol. Science *196*, 319—321 (1977)

197. Suntzeff, V., Burns, E. L., Moskop, M., Loeb, L.: On the proliferative changes taking place in the epithelium of vagina and cervix of mice with advancing age and under influence of experimentally administered estrogenic hormones. Am. J. Cancer *32*, 256—289 (1938)

198. Sweeney, E. C., Evans, D. J.: Hepatic lesions in patients treated with synthetic anabolic steroids. J. Clin. Pathol. *29*, 626—633 (1976)

199. Symmers, W. St. C.: Carcinoma of breast in trans-sexual individuals after surgical and hormonal interference with the primary and secondary sex characteristics. Br. Med. J. *2*, 83—85 (1968)

200. Tausk, M.: Pharmacology of Hormones. Stuttgart: Georg Thieme Publishers, 1975

201. Thomas, B. L.: Methadone-associated gynecomastia. New Engl. J. Med. *294*, 169 (1976)

202. Thompson, E. B.: The cellular actions of glucocorticoids in relation to human neoplasms. Curr. Top. Mol. Endocrinol. *4*, 114—132 (1976)

203. Tormey, D. C., Waalkes, T. P., Simon, R. M.: Biological markers in breast cancer. II. Clinical correlations with human chorionic gonadotropin. Cancer *39*, 2391—2396 (1977)

204. Veterans Administration Cooperative Urologic Research Group: Treatment and survival of patients with cancer of the prostate. Surg. Gynecol. Obstet. *124*, 1011—1017 (1967)

205. Vischer, E., Wittstein, A.: Enzymic transformation of steroids by microorganisms. In: Advances in Enzymology and Related Subjects of Biochem. New York: Interscience 1958, Vol. XX, p. 237

206. Wade, N.: Anabolic steroids: Doctors denounce them, but athletes are not listening. Science *176*, 1399—1403 (1972)

207. Watrous, R. M., Olsen, R. T.: Diethylstilbestrol in industry: A test for early detection as an aid in prevention. Am. Ind. Hyg. Assoc. J. *20*, 469—472 (1959)

208. Wilson, J. D.: Recent studies on the mechanism of action of testosterone. New Engl. J. Med. *287*, 1284—1291 (1972)

209. World Health Organization Information Bulletin on the Survey of Chemicals Being Tested for Carcinogenicity. No. 7. Lyon: IARC, 1978

210. Wynder, E. L., Mabuchi, K., Whitmore, W. F.: Epidemiology of cancer of the prostate. Cancer *28*, 344—360 (1971)

211. Zackheim, H. S.: Effect of castration of the induction of epidermal neoplasms in male mice by topical methylcholanthrene. J. Invest. Dermatol. *59*, 479—482 (1970)

212. Ziel, H. K., Finkle, W. D.: Increased risk of endometrial carcinoma among users of conjugated estrogens. New Engl. J. Med. *293*, 1167—1170 (1975)

213. Zumoff, B., Fishman, J., Cassouto, J., Hellman, L., Gallagher, T. F.: Estradiol transformation in men with breast cancer. J. Clin. Endocrinol. *26*, 960—966 (1966)

Pathologic Effects of Oral Contraceptives[1]

George D. Hilliard and Henry J. Norris

Much information has accumulated on the pathologic effects of oral contraceptive steroids. Many of the reports of untoward effects of oral contraceptives are anecdotal, but it is through the accumulation of isolated case studies that the impetus is given to initiate well-planned clinical and epidemiologic investigations, which in turn establish a scientific basis for any pathologic effects that have occurred. Oral contraceptives have been reported to cause abnormalities in organ systems of the liver (discussed in another paper in this monograph), cervix, endometrium, breast, ovary, vasculature, and in the complex systems of coagulation, renin-angiotensin, carbohydrate, and lipid metabolism, and also with endocrine interrelations. In this chapter, the organ systems will be discussed in turn; for the systemic effects, the reader will be referred to reviews.

Although many of the descriptions of pathologic abnormalities in oral contraceptive users are only case studies, enough information has accumulated to make it obvious that long-term study is needed of the effects of oral contraceptives. Women who take oral contraceptives should retain that information in their medical history even after they have stopped taking them, and a national registry should be organized to register women who die while taking oral contraceptives so that meaningful data can be accumulated. Screening measures should be undertaken in women taking oral contraceptives to detect early any undesirable side effects so that major complication can be averted. Women who plan to take oral contraceptives should first have a complete history and physical examination so that any abnormality can be identified that might predispose them to injury from using oral contraceptives.

Cervix

Oral contraceptives cause a mild, physiologic hyperplasia with increased secretion of the mucinous epithelium of the endocervix. Edema and decidual change may occur in the stroma. The higher the dose of the progestin, the more pronounced are the changes. The most abnormal finding is a distinctive polypoid endocervical hyperplasia [19, 62, 121, 130], termed microglandular hyperplasia. The lesion is a soft polyp, usually less than 1.5 cm in diameter, and consists of a dense agglomeration of glands and tubules of varying sizes composed of flat, cuboidal, or columnar cells (Fig. 1). The cells are uniform, but some have slightly hyperchromatic nuclei. Usually there is an accompanying inflammatory infiltrate. Patients with this lesion are usually clinically asymptomatic but may have postcoital or intermenstrual spotting. The microglandular hyperplasia is sufficiently specific that it is easily recognized microscopi-

---

1 The opinions or assertions contained herein are the private views of the authors and are not to be construed as official or as reflecting the views of the Department of the Army, of the Air Force, or of Defense.

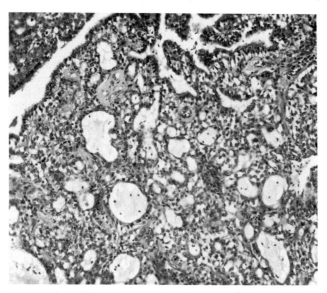

Fig. 1. Microglandular hyperplasia of the cervix ("pill polyp") in a woman taking an oral contraceptive. In the early years of oral contraceptive usage, this lesion was sometimes misinterpreted as carcinoma. AFIP Neg. No. 75-7656, H & E, × 115

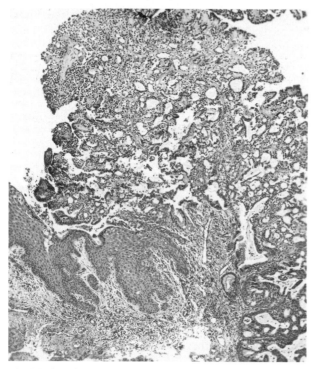

Fig. 2. Microglandular hyperplasia superimposed on adenosis of the vagina in a young woman using an oral contraceptive who was exposed to diethylstilbestrol in utero. Reports of this lesion in adenosis of the vagina have sometimes been confused with adenocarcinoma. AFIP Neg. No. 77-5252, H & E, × 50

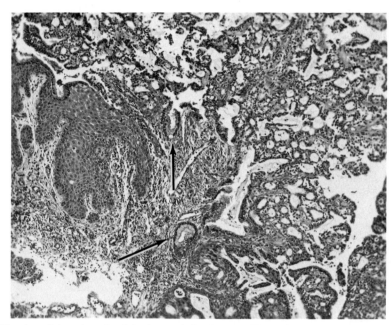

Fig. 3. Higher magnification of the microglandular hyperplasia shown in Figure 2. *Arrows* point to the underyling mucinous endocervical type of glands. AFIP Neg. No. 77-5251, H & E, × 70

cally, and it is seldom confused with carcinoma. A smaller but similar microscopic finding can be found in some pregnant patients. It does not occur in elderly women receiving estrogenic substances, and thus progesterone is the common denominator in the pathogenesis of microglandular hyperplasia. Microglandular hyperplasia of the endocervix is reversible upon cessation of the oral contraceptive agent. Although 5% of patients do not have a record of oral contraceptive use or recent pregnancy, the negative histories are not reliable, as they do not mean the women were not taking them. The fully developed polypoid lesion was not encountered in the absence of pregnancy prior to the advent of oral contraceptives. KURMAN and NORRIS [60] pointed out that microglandular hyperplasia is now encountered in the vagina, superimposed on an underlying adenosis (Figs. 2 and 3) in users of oral contraceptives who had in utero exposure to stilbestrol [95]. Unfortunately, two or three examples appear to have been misinterpreted as cancer [46, 60].

Abnormal cervical cytology [29, 58, 64, 65, 74, 75], intraepithelial neoplasia, and cervical carcinoma [25] were reported to have increased in patients using oral contraceptive steroids, but there is no evidence that the contraceptives are responsible for the finding [8, 16, 100]. There is a higher rate of cervical atypia among women who choose oral steroids for contraception over those who choose another means of contraception [74, 75, 117]. It may be that pill users are more sexually active [65, 80] and the abnormal cervical cytology present prior to selection of the oral contraceptive can be explained on the basis of the venereal characteristics of cervical squamous neoplasia. Some reports fail to detect a difference in the sexual habits of patients on the oral contraceptives [38], however, and not all studies support the findings of increased cervical abnormalities in patients after oral contraceptive therapy [8, 16, 104]. Studies show that in some public clinics women who select oral contraceptive agents have an increase in cervical intraepithelial neoplasia [74, 75, 83, 117]. No studies show that pill users are more likely to develop an increase in cervical neoplasia, although a recent statistical evaluation suggests that dysplasias progress more rapidly in women taking oral contraceptives than in controls [117].

Endometrium

The effect of oral contraceptives on the endometrium is related to the components of the drug and the dose used [35, 44, 70, 79, 81]. The effect varies, depending on whether the regimen is a combination, sequential, or purely progestational. All of these drugs affect only the functional portion of the endometrium. The basalis remains unresponsive to endogenous or exogenous steroids.

The combination regimen has a fixed amount of estrogen and progestin in each tablet. The regimen begins on day 5 of the cycle or the last day of anticipated bleeding and continues for

Table 1. Effects of oral contraceptive agents on the endometrium

Combined regimen	Day of cycle	Sequential regimen
Take pill No. 1	5	Take first of 14 estrogen pills
	6	
Little or no glandular development	7	
	8	
	9	
Subnuclear vacuoles apear	10	
	11	
Glands gradually disappear	12	
Large stroma/gland ratio	13	Glands develop as usual
	14	
Variable degree of supranuclear vacuoles	15	
	16	
	17	
	18	
	19	Begin estrogen and progestin pill
	20	
Regression of secretory changes	21	Subnuclear vacuoles appear
	22	Atrophy of gland optional
	23	Stroma/gland ratio approximately normal
	24	
Stop pills	25	Stop pills
Decidual changes appear in most (endometrium thin with repeated cycles)	26	Decidual change optional: secretory glands present
	27	
Bleeding starts (less than usual)	28	Bleeding starts (approximately normal)

20–21 days. The progestin dominates, inhibiting glandular growth but inducing subnuclear vacuoles, which appear early — after only 5 days of administration (day 10 of the cycle) (Table 1; Fig. 4). The stroma is relatively inactive, the glands are not just inhibited but may gradually disappear, and by day 20 of the cycle there is an increased stroma-to-gland ratio [9, 79, 81, 97, 98, 99]. The secretory effects are mild and transient, depending on the dose of progestin. The endometrium becomes thinner with repeated cycles, and withdrawal of medication provokes less bleeding than the usual because it is thin. Endothelial hyperplasia may occur within endometrial capillaries and arterioles, and there may be thrombosis or fibrin plugs in dilated endometrial vessels [51, 79, 81, 108]. The spiral arterioles do not develop [57, 80, 81].

Sequential oral contraceptives were designated "sequential" because the regimen consists of estrogen for the first 14–16 days, followed sequentially by 4–6 days of estrogen combined with progestin. No longer available in the United States [31], the sequential regimen produces a period of 14–16 days of unopposed estrogen stimulation. The addition of a progestin to the estrogen on day 19 or 20 of the cycle inhibits further proliferation of the glands. Subnuclear vacuoles appear in 2 days (Table 1); after 4–6 days of the estrogen-progestin combination, secretory and usually decidual changes appear. A bleeding phase follows withdrawal of the drug. The sequential regimen is slightly less effective than the combined regimen in preventing pregnancy [26]. There is a greater likelihood of endometrial hyperplasia with the sequential steroid oral contraceptives since there are 14–16 days of unopposed estrogen. A summary of the cyclic endometrial changes occurring with the combined and sequential regimens is shown in Table 1.

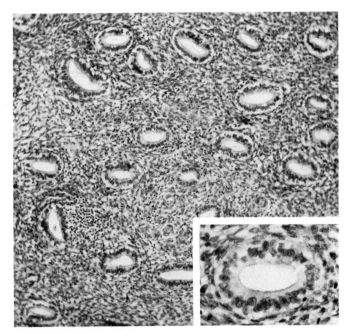

Fig. 4. Endometrium on the 10th day of the cycle and the 5th day of a combined oral contraceptive. Insert shows the characteristic subnuclear vacuoles. AFIP Neg. No. 77-4783, H & E, × 100. Insert AFIP Neg. No. 77-4784, H & E, × 265

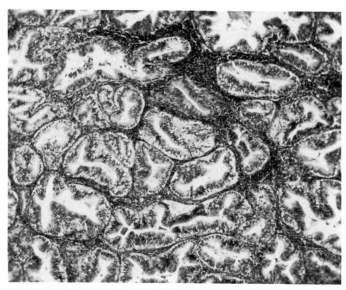

Fig. 5. Endometrial hyperplasia with a secretory effect from a patient who had been taking a sequential oral contraceptive 2 years. AFIP Neg. No. 77-5254, H & E, × 100

The pattern of the endometrium with progestins continuously administered in "microdoses" (minipills) is more variable but occasionally may be similar to that in patients receiving the combination regimen [76, 77], although there is more of a decidual reaction. Since ovulation occurs in approximately three-quarters of patients receiving microdose progestins [77], the histologic pattern of the endometrium is variable, depending on the type and dosage of the progestational agent in use [44, 97] — whether it is a 19-nortestosterone or a 17α-hydroxyprogesterone derivative (the latter is excluded from present-day pills). There is an increased stroma-to-gland ratio, as there is inhibition of glands. Stromal edema, decidual reaction, and increased stromal cellularity tend to occur. These changes probably impede implantation of the ovum, but continuous microdose progestins prevent conception also through their actions on the cervical mucus and altered hypothalamic function as well as alteration of the histologic pattern of the endometrium. Irregular and unpredictable vaginal bleeding is a common side effect when the microdose progestins are used [77], but for those women who have side effects related to synthetic estrogens, the progestins may help alleviate them.

Endometrial hyperplasia and carcinoma have been reported in women taking oral contraceptive steroids [54, 55, 67, 68, 105, 106]. The sequential regimen was associated with carcinoma more commonly than expected from its use in the general population. This could have been anticipated, as the sequential regimen is estrogen dominated, exerts a transient hyperplasia in some women, and would not be expected to inhibit an endometrium predisposed to carcinoma. Of 21 young women taking oral contraceptives who developed endometrial carcinoma [105], nine had well-differentiated adenocarcinoma; two had mixed adenosquamous carcinoma; one, a clear cell (mesonephroid) carcinoma; and three had adenocarcinoma exhibiting a marked secretory effect. In two other instances, the adenocarcinomas had a focal secretory pattern. The secretory activity was attributed to the progestational component of the oral contraceptive. The common finding of a squamous component in these neoplasms is not surprising, since about half of endometrial adenocarcinomas exhibit this feature and estrogen

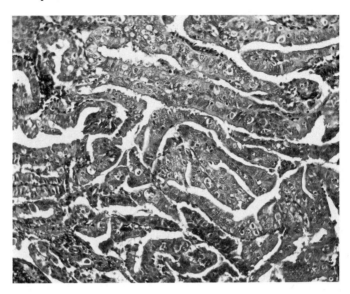

Fig. 6. Endometrial carcinoma from a 33-year-old woman who had been taking a sequential oral contraceptive for 2 years. AFIP Neg. No. 77-4770, H & E, × 130

is thought possibly to promote the occurrence of squamous metaplasia in endometrial carcinoma. Endometrial samples from patients on sequential oral contraceptives are shown in Figures 5 and 6.

There is no relationship between endometrial carcinoma and the combined regimen, and in view of the inhibitory effect of the regimen on endometrial glands, hyperplasia is not likely to occur [44, 57]. The Arias-Stella reaction has been rarely reported with ordinary doses of some steroidal contraceptive drugs [9, 108]. Endometrial stromal sarcoma has been reported in patients taking the combination oral contraceptives [108], but the documentation is dubious.

Myometrium

Estrogen induces the myometrial cells to undergo hyperplasia and hypertrophy in some animal species, whereas progesterone tends to enhance the estrogen effect of an estrogen-primed uterus [71, 93]. This response to both steroids varies from one species to another as well as with the distensibility of the uterus and dose of the steroid [71]. There was no change in the uterine size of six patients who received a combined oral contraceptive steroid for 1 year and were studied clinically with ultrasound [89].

There are claims that oral contraceptives affect leiomyomas in two ways: (1) by producing nuclear atypism in some instances [32, 43, 92] and (2) by producing hemorrhagic degeneration of abnormally cellular foci [9, 43] (Fig. 7). Nuclear abnormalities occur spontaneously in the absence of steroids, and there is no experimental basis for this feature. The mitotic activity of these leiomyomas is low; therefore, the finding has no malignant potential. Hemorrhagic degeneration in leiomyomas occurs mainly in women taking oral contraceptives but is rare in the absence of steroids. Hemorrhagic degeneration probably begins with central edema,

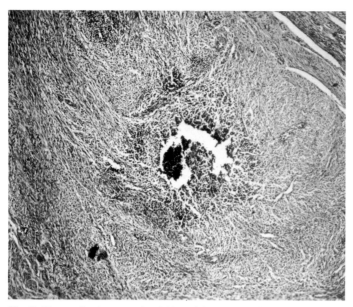

Fig. 7. Hemorrhagic necrosis within a leiomyoma of the uterus in a patient taking a combined oral contraceptive. This form of hemorrhage within a leiomyoma is strongly associated with oral contraceptives. AFIP Neg. No. 76-7386, H & E, × 52

followed by hemorrhage, which in turn leads to necrosis and subsequent scarring [43]. Mitotic activity may be common around hemorrhagic foci, prompting confusion with leiomyosarcoma. The steroid history and multifocal aspect of the hemorrhage should prompt closer inspection, however. Fatty degeneration, fibrosis, and hyalinization have also been described with the use of progestin [43]. Perhaps the initial edema and hemorrhage produce an increase in the size of myomas [32], while long-term therapy contributes to a delay of growth because of hyalinization resulting from scarring in areas of hemorrhage. There is no agreement on whether or not progestins are useful as therapy for leiomyomas.

Fallopian Tube

During the menstrual cycle, morphologic changes are not consistently visible at the light-microscopic level of examination. Even by transmission and scanning electron microscopy, morphologic changes vary from study to study [76]. A partial listing of the inconsistent cyclic changes that have been reported to occur in the fallopian tube can be found elsewhere [18]. Thus, it is not surprising that there is disagreement on whether or not cyclic changes in the epithelium of the fallopian tube are under the influence of oral contraceptives. The reported effects of oral contraceptives can be summarized as follows:
1. Estrogens stimulate ciliated cells to produce cilia, whereas progestins inhibit this growth [82];
2. There is epithelial hyperplasia by increased secretory and indifferent cells and by an increase in the number of enlarged epithelial cells [44];
3. Combined preparations of oral contraceptives and progestins may cause focal increases in the height of the epithelium, enlargement of nuclei, and loss of cilia [37, 85];

4. Mild alterations of the epithelium occur in the infundibulum rather than in the ampulla [37];

5. Tubal motility and ciliary activity decrease with combined agents, although they increase with estrogen alone [14]. A decidual reaction is sometimes observed in the serosal and mucosal layers of the fallopian tube with exogenous progestin therapy. The alteration occurs under the influence of the reproductive steroids and generally involves the subserosal and mucosal layers.

Ovary

Oral contraceptive steroids inhibit ovulation. This inhibition occurs through the suppression of the synthesis or release of pituitary gonadotropins [28, 36]. Estrogen inhibits follicle-stimulating hormone (FSH) production; progestin suppresses the mid cycle surge of luteinizing hormone (LH). Progestin and estrogen in the combined regimen probably inhibit secretion of hypothalamic releasing factors [114]. Progestins, through a negative feedback action on the hypothalamus, inhibit secretion of hypothalamic releasing factors. Estrogens enhance this negative (inhibitory) feedback effect of the progestins. The low-dose oral contraceptive steroids may not inhibit ovulation, and of those that do, some are intermittently suppressive [70, 82, 131].

Histologic examination of the ovary in patients taking combined oral contraceptive steroids shows that the number and appearance of oocytes are unaffected. The follicles tend to be inactive and of a uniform size, usually small, and a corpus luteum is not usually present, although one may be present if the patient had "break-through" ovulation. The follicles that have formed antra do not have a luteinized theca interna [70].In some cases the outer cortical stroma may appear condensed or fibrous [70, 90, 99, 133], since it — similarly to the follicles — is not stimulated. The appearance is that of an inactive ovary and the changes disappear with restoration of normal pituitary function.

Persistent anovulation in young women following use of the oral contraceptive steroids has been designated the "ovarian suppression syndrome". A better term is "hypothalamic suppression", because the syndrome results from inhibition of hypothalamic releasing factors and a resulting decrease in gonadotropin release from the pituitary. Amenorrhea after discontinuing the oral contraceptive occurs only twice per 1000 women and does not appear to correlate with the duration of the oral steroids [42]. After discontinuance, 98% of patients resume ovulation and will have normal endometrial function with the first three cycles [94, 116]. The frequency of the "ovarian suppression syndrome" is no higher than the frequency of anovulatory women in the population at large, and it is uncertain if it results from use of oral contraceptives, since a control study has not been done. Nevertheless, many clinicians recommend that only women with proven fertility be given oral contraceptives. If amenorrhea is found in a patient with galactorrhea after oral contraceptive therapy, the possibility of a pituitary adenoma or endocrinologic dysfunction should be investigated [39, 42, 116, 123]. An association between the use of oral contraceptives and pituitary adenomas has not yet been demonstrated.

Vagina

The sequential regimens and the combined regimens containing higher doses of estrogen (estrogen-dominated) induce cornification of the vaginal mucosa. Some combination preparations that are progestin dominated tend to inhibit cornification of the vaginal mucosa and produce an increased susceptibility to infection [52, 73]. Although some women on oral contraceptives complain of a vaginal discharge, this is usually watery and secondary to increased mucus secretion of the glandular epithelium of the cervix rather than from a vaginitis. Vaginitis in patients receiving the oral contraceptive steroids is often monilial. In one study, the finding of monilial vaginitis was 15% in users of oral contraceptives and 5% in nonusers [53]. The increase in susceptibility of the vagina to *Monilia* is probably due to incomplete cornification of the vaginal mucosa or to alteration in local carbohydrate metabolism or to both. Moniliasis may be quite extensive, involving the vulva as well. In a cross-sectional study by SPELLACY et al. [113], however, the frequency of positive yeast cultures for patients using intrauterine devices did not differ significantly from those using sequential oral contraceptives or combination drugs. In a prospective study cultures were taken from similar groups of patients and no significant differences were observed in the frequency of *Candida albicans* vaginitis, or blood glucose, or plasma insulin in patients with or without positive yeast cultures.

In patients with vaginal adenosis who receive oral contraceptives, microglandular hyperplasia may develop in areas of adenosis [60, 95] (Fig. 2). These polypoid benign growths may be confused with adenocarcinoma if the pathologist is not given the history of contraceptive usage.

Breast

The breast is under the influence of endogenous ovarian steroids during the menstrual cycle as well as prolactin and growth hormone synthesized and released by the pituitary gland. Insulin, thyroxin, and cortisol must also be available for full differentiation of the mammary gland. The growth of ductal epithelium and maintenance of the stroma of the breast is largely via estrogen, whereas progesterone promotes growth and development of lobules and acini and induces secretory activity [63, 114].

Atypical epithelial proliferation and carcinomas occur in women taking oral contraceptive steroids, but there is currently no evidence to support the contention that the drugs have a causal relationship in their development. In fact, a survey of the Boston Collaborative Drug Surveillance Program suggested that the use of oral contraceptives may have a protective effect against the development of benign breast lesions [15]. Control studies have not shown an increase in mammary cancer in oral contraceptive users, nor have most patients with breast cancer used oral contraceptives.

There is speculation about the long-term effect of contraceptive steroids on the breast. The inhibitory effect on the pituitary may secondarily affect functional and structural components of breast tissue, but this is counteracted by the effect of the estrogens and progestins directly on mammary tissue. It is not known if oral contraceptives contribute to the development of benign lesions, atypical hyperplasia, or malignant neoplasms. The finding of mammary nodules in beagles receiving chlormadinone [78] added to the concern, but it is doubtful that abnormalities induced by steroids in the beagle can be extrapolated to women, since the beagle is uniquely susceptible to progestins and the type of nodules that develop in beagles are very rare in women.

The histologic changes found in the normal breasts of some women receiving oral contraceptives are (1) a focal or diffuse increase in lobular development by dilatation and possibly proliferation of acini; (2) an enlargement of acinar cells with secretory changes; and (3) edema of the intralobular stroma [33, 35]. Secretion tends to collect in acinar lumens and small ducts. These findings are variable and not seen in all patients [120]. The changes are not specific for patients receiving oral contraceptives, since they are similar to those found in pregnant and lactating women (Figs. 8—11).

GOLDENBERG et al. [41] described epithelial hyperplasia in fibroadenomas in women taking oral contraceptives. Although no one believed that the oral contraceptives caused the fibroadenomas, observers thought that the steroids were possibly responsible for a florid epithelial proliferation within the fibroadenomas. In contrast, FECHNER [33] found no distinctive features (or epithelial hyperplasia) in fibroadenomas in women receiving oral contraceptives as compared with age-matched controls not taking contraceptive steroids. FECHNER did find some degree of acinar hyperplasia in four nulligravid women that was possibly a result of the contraceptives. In a second study [34] FECHNER found no histologic changes within fibrocystic disease that could be attributed to oral contraceptives. Thus, at present there is no firm association between the development of benign breast neoplasms and use of oral contraceptives [7, 35, 63, 101, 118, 120, 126, 127]. Contraceptive steroids have been utilized in therapy of clinical fibrocystic disease [6], but it is not clear if they have any value. Some patients report tenderness, fullness, and even an increase in the size of their breasts while taking oral contraceptives. When these symptoms occur, it is with the initial use, and after several cycles most of the complaints subside. Occasionally, because of symptoms, there may be a need either to switch preparations or discontinue their use altogether.

Some patients taking oral contraceptives, particularly the higher doses of estrogenic pills, develop galactorrhea, probably resulting from a disorder of pituitary prolactin secretion [63, 123]. Other important factors in this galactorrhea are probably related to the increased lobular development and proliferation of acini [35].

Carcinomas of the breast with unusual features have been reported to develop in women taking oral contraceptives [45, 87]. The oral steroids did not have a causal relationship in the induction of the carcinomas because the duration of usage was too short in a disease with the doubling time of breast cancer averaging 25 days [86]. With average doubling times, it takes at least 2 years after induction before a neoplasm will become clinically evident. KUSAMA et al. [61] have found that tumor-doubling times are shorter and therefore rates of growth more rapid in young women (21—30 years of age). These investigators, as well as GERSHON-COHEN et al. [40], have found somewhat different doubling times (40—200 days) for breast carcinomas. Concern over the possibility of oral contraceptives' role in the development of breast carcinoma resulted from (1) reports of persons taking estrogen who develop carcinoma; (2) an unusual modification of the course of their disease in women while taking steroids; and (3) examples of neoplasms developing in several animal species taking steroids. A monkey developed mammary carcinoma after taking Enovid (norethynodrel) for 18 months [56], but DRILL et al. [30] found no clinical evidence of mammary gland lesions in 96 rhesus monkeys treated with Enovid-E and Ovulen for 5 years. PENMAN [87] described an unusual histologic effect within mammary carcinoma, including large foamy atypical cells that he felt were colostrum cells, along with a marked secretory change in the breast of a 27-year-old woman receiving oral contraceptives who was found to have an infiltrating mammary carcinoma. GOULD et al. [45] also reported similar alterations in the ducts and lobules of breast carcinomas in patients taking oral contraceptives, apparently a modification of the tumor by steroids. These two reports serve as a warning that if a steroid can modify the histologic appearance of mammary cancers in rare instances, then it may also alter the growth rate and perhaps serve as a cocarcinogen in rare instances. At present there is no other evidence that oral contraceptives induce mammary cancer or atypical hyperplasia.

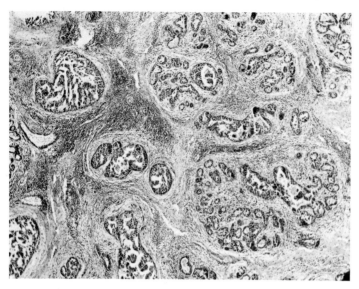

Fig. 8. Biopsy from the breast of a patient taking an oral contraceptive steroid. Lobules (*right*) and ducts (*left*) show markedly atypical alterations. Prominent lymphoid stroma is also present. AFIP Neg. No. 77-5619, H & E, × 35

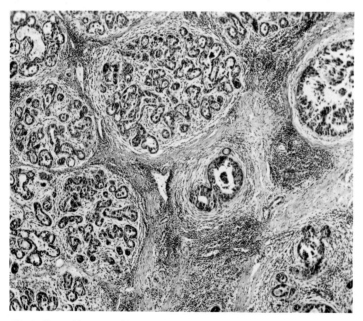

Fig. 9. Same biopsy as Figure 8 showing lobules lined by atypical cells and dilated acini containing a secretory product, presumably a steroid effect. AFIP Neg. No. 77-5591, H & E, × 63

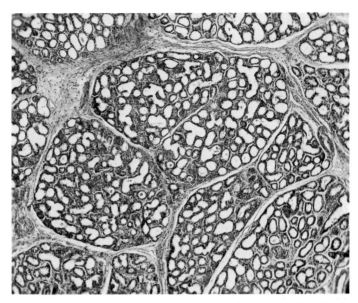

Fig. 10. Same breast biopsy as shown in Figures 8 and 9. Note marked lactational effect in the otherwise normal lobule. This degree of lobular hyperplasia is not seen in the absence of hormone stimulation by nursing, pregnancy, oral contraceptives, or certain nonsteroidal galactogenic stimulants to the central nervous system. AFIP Neg. No. 77-5594, H & E, × 56

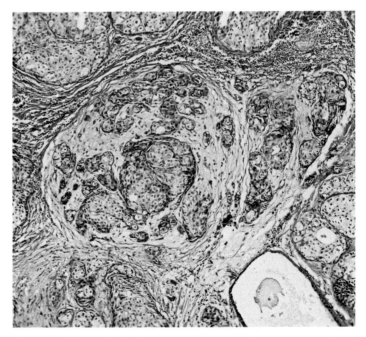

Fig. 11. This carcinoma from the breast of a patient taking an oral contraceptive shows a prominent myxoid stroma, apparently an estrogen effect. AFIP Neg. No. 77-5727, H & E, × 77

Thrombosis

The frequency of thrombosis has increased three—fivefold in women using oral contraceptive steroids over that of a population of women the same age not taking them [49, 102, 124, 125]. Alterations in coagulation have received much attention [2, 4, 13, 17], but direct vascular injury in women taking oral contraceptives has also been reported [50, 84]. In 1970, IREY et al. [51] found vascular lesions in 20 women who had taken combined and sequential oral contraceptive steroids. Vascular lesions, found in arteries and veins of the pulmonary system and portal circulation apart from sites of thrombosis, consisted of cellular intimal proliferation, a fibrous intimal proliferation, and a peculiar myxoid alteration. IREY and NORRIS [50] subsequently described vascular lesions in 16 women who were pregnant, postpartum, or using oral contraceptives. Five women were pregnant and in their second or third trimester. The sites of the vascular lesions were arteries of the lung, kidney, heart, liver, intestines, adrenal, uterus, and vulva. Four postpartum patients had vascular lesions in their coronary and renal arteries. Seven patients received oral contraceptives. The duration of use varied from 6 weeks to 5 years. The lesions were found in arteries of mesentery, lung, cervix, and inguinal areas. Hepatic and mesenteric veins were also involved. Microscopically, all vascular lesions were characterized by intimal proliferation, most of which was very cellular, with very little intervening stroma. Several lesions were associated with an overlying thrombus. Narrowing of the lumen resulted in myocardial infarction, myocardial fibrosis, and mesenteric infarction and contributed to pulmonary hypertension and renal failure. Similar intimal lesions were found in patients of two control groups. The first control group, consisting of 40 women who had died suddenly from various illnesses included two patients with intimal thickening and luminal narrowing, but one of these patients was found upon investigation to have been taking an oral contraceptive containing mestranol and norethynodrel. In a second group of 67 control patients dying from a variety of cardiovascular diseases, similar intimal lesions were seen. Therefore the lesions are not specific for steroid users, but they do occur in

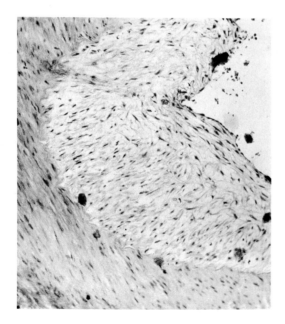

Fig. 12. Myxoid fibrous intimal thickening of a branch of a mesenteric artery in a patient taking an oral contraceptive for 5 years. AFIP Neg. No. 70-4552. (Used with Irey, N. S., Norris, H. J.: Intimal vascular lesions associated with female reproductive steroids. Arch. Pathol. *96*, 227, Oct. 1973. Copyright 1973, American Medical Association), H & E, × 115

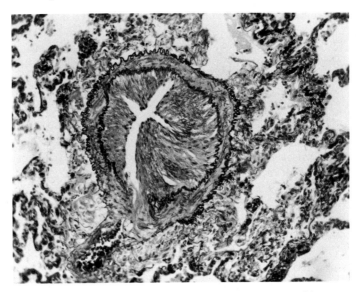

Fig. 13. Lumen is narrowed from intimal proliferation in the pulmonary artery of a 29-year-old woman taking an oral contraceptive. AFIP Neg. No. 70-8875. (Irey, N. S., Norris, H. J.: Intimal vascular lesions associated with female reproductive steroids. Arch. Pathol. *96*, 227, Oct. 1973. Copyright 1973, American Medical Association), Movat's pentachrome, × 195

patients using oral contraceptives who do not have known or preexisting cardiovascular disease. WAGONER et al. [128] and ROBSON et al. [96], in separate reports, described intimal thickening and proliferation of renal arteries in women with postpartum renal failure. Vascular lesions can be induced in guinea pigs by estrogen, providing an experimental model for study. OSTERHOLZER et al. [84] recently examined the uteri from women who took oral contraceptives before undergoing hysterectomy. Compared with a control population, they found moderate (less than 50% occlusion) or severe (50% or greater cross-sectional luminal occlusion) intimal proliferation in 31 of 38 patients who had used contraceptives.

Female reproductive steroids act to induce intimal proliferation, which in turn reduces the lumen of the vessel. This, in combination with altered coagulation, may result in symptoms. Figures 12 and 13 illustrate several effects of oral contraceptive steroids on vessels.

Thromboembolic Disease

Some women receiving oral contraceptives showed an increase in (1) superficial venous thrombosis, (2) thrombosis of deep veins, (3) pulmonary embolism, and (4) cerebral ischemia and thrombosis [21, 22, 49, 102].

VESSEY and DOLL [125] reported a ninefold increase in hospital admissions for venous thromboembolism in patients taking oral contraceptives, as compared with nonusers. SARTWELL et al. [102] found the risk of thromboembolism in oral contraceptive users to be about four times higher than that of those who did not take oral contraceptives, and the risk was highest in women taking sequential agents. The duration of use did not affect the risk. Estrogen is thought to be the component mainly responsible for alterations of the clotting mechanism. The combination oral contraceptives in susceptible persons enhance blood coagulation and increase platelet aggregation, certain clotting factors, and fibrinolysis [2, 4, 13, 17]. Thrombosis may result from a failure of the normal fibrinolytic mechanism or from increased lability of the clotting system. The reader is referred to reviews of the relationship between oral contraceptives and thromboembolism [2, 21, 22, 49, 102, 103, 124, 125].

Hypertension

Oral contraceptives may induce hypertension or exacerbate preexisting hypertension through alteration of the renin-angiotensin system. Other important alterations may occur in renal sodium and water handling and the sympathetic nervous system. Estrogen causes a marked elevation of plasma angiotensinogen (renin substrate) [10, 66, 119]. Renin acts on this substrate to produce angiotensin I, which is hydrolyzed to produce angiotensin II, an active pressor substance. Angiotensin II stimulates the adrenal cortex to produce aldosterone, which causes water and sodium retention. This, along with variables such as blood volume and increased arteriolar tone, may produce hypertension, especially if there is increased cardiac output and a compensatory failure of sodium and water excretion. The estrogen component of oral contraceptives appears to be the main agent responsible for hypertension, but the progestin component has not been completely absolved [24]. It is not possible to explain the elevation of blood pressure on the renin-angiotensin system alone. Plasma renin substrate and plasma renin activity are increased in both hypertensive and normotensive patients on oral contraceptives [10, 66, 119]. Plasma renin concentrations have not been consistently increased or decreased in all studies [10] in patients receiving oral contraceptive steroids. It has been postulated that in normotensive users of oral contraceptives, renin levels are low because angiotensin prevents renin release through a negative feedback mechanism on the kidney [10]. Evidence is also available of significantly reduced plasma renin concentrations, however, in both hypertensive and normotensive women on oral contraceptives [10, 66]. It appears that a failure of the inhibitory effect of high levels of angiotensin on renin release (negative feedback) is not the only explanation for development of hypertension in users of oral contraceptives. When hypertension occurs, it is usually within the first 6 months. Both diastolic and systolic levels may be elevated. Usually the blood pressure returns to normal levels within 3–6 months after cessation of oral contraceptive therapy [10, 66, 107]. Although the hypertension is usually mild, there are rare reports of hypertensive crises and renal failure in patients receiving contraceptive steroids [122, 132].

BERAL [11] recently published data concerning cardiovascular and cerebrovascular disease mortality and oral contraceptive use for women 15–44 years old from 21 countries through the World Health Organization reports. Through statistical analysis of mortality trends he found a "clear relationship between oral contraceptive use and changes in mortality rates from nonrheumatic heart disease and hypertension, cerebrovascular disease, and all nonrheumatic cardiovascular diseases" over a 10-year period. The estimated relative risks of death for these three categories of women who took oral contraceptives as compared to nonusers were 5 to 1, 2 to 1, and 3 to 1, respectively.

Carbohydrate Metabolism

Oral contraceptive steroids may decrease glucose tolerance. This finding is more apparent in women who are latent or overt diabetics or who have a family history of diabetes, obesity, or delivery of a large infant or unexplained stillbirth [111]. Patients taking oral contraceptives have increased plasma insulin levels and an increase in peripheral resistance to the action of insulin. Other properties of oral contraceptives that influence carbohydrate metabolism include alteration in liver function influencing gluconeogenesis and glycogenolysis, elevation of levels of human growth hormone by estrogen, elevation of the cortisol level, alteration of metabolism of tryptophan, and a decrease in pyridoxine [110]. Some women show a transient decrease in glucose tolerance, which may return to premedication tolerance values while they are still receiving the drug (probably patients who can increase their insulin production). POSNER et al. [91] found a prompt and significant decline in glucose tolerance in nondiabetic subjects and in a group suspected of being latent diabetics during long-term oral contraceptive therapy. In one study the mean blood glucose levels in women receiving oral contraceptives was 11 mg/100 ml higher than in nonusers of oral contraceptives [88]. SPELLACY [111] found increases in both the blood glucose levels and plasma insulin values for patients receiving oral contraceptives. Progestins are mainly responsible for producing alterations in carbohydrate metabolism, although estrogen may act synergistically with progestin [112]. Estrogen, when given to premenopausal women, has little effect on carbohydrate metabolism [111].

Carbohydrate abnormalities subside when oral contraceptives are discontinued. Ideally, patients at risk for diabetes mellitus should be identified before prescribing of oral contraceptives.

Other metabolic effects of oral contraceptives are an increase in serum cholesterol and triglycerides [111], phospholipids, and fatty acids [3]. These effects are variable, however. The net effect of the metabolic changes on the cardiovascular system is unknown. Long-term studies will be needed to learn if atherosclerosis is increased in patients taking oral contraceptives.

Summary

The pathologic effects of oral contraceptives have been described in this paper and in other reviews [1, 5, 23, 35, 44, 48, 59, 80, 103, 114].

Approximately 10 million women currently use oral contraceptives in the United States. These drugs are beneficial both to the users and for population control. It is their effect on the health status of women who take them that must continue to have well-organized investigation so that more meaningful conclusions concerning their safety will permit continued use. In some instances, the pathologic effects of oral contraceptives make it necessary that new methods of contraception be found. Intensive research in this area is needed and judicious use of oral contraceptives must be maintained.

A national registry should be formed to record and investigate the cases of women who die or have adverse reactions while taking these agents. A registry might identify associations no previously known to exist in patients taking oral contraceptives. It would serve to concentrate the data in one area so that more material would be available for the study of pathogenetic mechanisms. It would heighten patient and physician awareness of the untoward effects and increase the responsibilities of the women who take them to monitor their own health.

References

1. ACOG Technical Bulletin Number *41*. Oral contraception (1976)
2. Alkjaersig, N., Fletcher, A., Burstein, R.: Association between oral contraceptive use and thromboembolism: A new approach to its investigation based on plasma fibrinogen chromatography. Am. J. Obstet. Gynecol. *122*, 199–211 (1975)

3. De Alvarez, R. R., Jahed, F. M., Spitalny, K. J., Elkin, H., Jaunakais, I.: The influence of oral contraceptive steroids on serum lipids. Am. J. Obstet. Gynecol. *116*, 727—749 (1973)
4. Ambrus, J. L., Mink, I. B., Courey, N. G., Niswander, K., Moore, R. H., Ambrus, C. M., Lillie, M. A.: Progestational agents and blood coagulation. VII. Thromboembolic and other complications of oral contraceptive therapy in relationship to pretreatment levels of blood coagulation factors: Summary report of a ten-year study. Am. J. Obstet. Gynecol. *125*, 1057—1062 (1976)
5. Andrews, W. C.: Oral contraception: a review of reported physiological and pathological effects. Obstet. Gynecol. Surv. *26*, 477—499 (1971)
6. Ariel, I. M.: Enovid therapy (norethynodrel with mestranol) for fibrocystic disease. Am. J. Obstet. Gynecol. *117*, 453—459 (1973)
7. Arthes, F. G., Sartwell, P. E., Lewison, E. F.: The pill, estrogens and the breast: epidemiologic aspects. Cancer *28*, 1391—1394 (1971)
8. Ayre, J. E., Hillemanns, H. G., Leguerrier, J., Arsenault, J.: Influence of norethynodrel and mestranol upon cervical dysplasia and carcinoma in situ. Obstet. Gynecol. *28*, 90—98 (1966)
9. Azzopardi, J. G., Zayid, I.: Synthetic progestogen-oestrogen therapy and uterine changes. J. Clin. Pathol. *20*, 731—738 (1967)
10. Beckerhoff, R., Luetscher, J. A., Wilkinson, R., Gonzales, C., Nokes, G. W.: Plasma renin concentration, activity, and substrate in hypertension induced by oral contraceptives. J. Clin. Endocrinol. Metab. *34*, 1067—1073 (1972)
11. Beral, V.: Cardiovascular disease mortality trends and oral contraceptive use in young women. Lancet *2*, 1047—1052 (1976)
12. Berge, B. S. ten: Histological changes in ovarian and uterine blood vessels after the use of oral contraceptive agents (estrogen-gestagen combinations) and gestagens. Int. J. Fertil. *18*, 57—63 (1973)
13. Bick, R. L., Thompson, W. B.: Fibrinolytic activity: changes induced with oral contraceptives. Obstet. Gynecol. *39*, 213—217 (1972)
14. Boling, J. L.: Endocrinology of oviductal musculature. In: The Mammalian Oviduct: Comparative Biology and Methodology. Hafez, E. S. E., Blandau, R. J. (Eds.). Chicago: The University of Chicago Press 1969, pp. 163—181
15. Boston Collaborative Drug Surveillance Program. Oral contraceptives and venous thromboembolic disease. Surgically confirmed gallbladder disease and breast tumors. Lancet *1*, 1399—1404 (1973)
16. Boyce, J. G., Lu, T., Nelson, J. H., Joyce, D.: Cervical carcinoma and oral contraception. Obstet. Gynecol. *40*, 139—146 (1972)
17. Brakman, P., Albrecktsen, O. K., Astrup, T.: Blood coagulation, fibrinolysis and contraceptive hormones. JAMA *199*, 69—74 (1967)
18. Brenner, R. M.: The biology of oviductal cilia. In: The Mammalian Oviduct: Comparative Biology and Methodology. Hafez, E. S. E., Blandau, R. J. (Eds.). Chicago: The University of Chicago Press, 1969, pp. 203—229
19. Candy, J., Abell, M. R.: Progestogen-induced hyperplasia of the cervix. JAMA *203*, 323—326 (1968)
20. Cohen, C. J., Deppe, G.: Endometrial carcinoma and oral contraceptive agents. Obstet. Gynecol. *49*, 390—392 (1977)
21. Collaborative Group for the Study of Stroke in Young Women: Oral contraception and increased risk of cerebral ischemia or thrombosis. New. Engl. J. Med. *288*, 871—878 (1973)
22. Comhaire, F., Vandeweghe, M., Vermeulen, A.: Vascular incidents and oral contraceptives: arterial versus venous thromboembolism: a statistical study. Contraception *3*, 301—312 (1971)
23. Craig, J. M.: The pathology of birth control. Arch. Pathol. *99*, 233—236 (1975)
24. Crane, M. G., Harris, J. J.: Plasma renin activity and aldosterone excretion rate in normal subjects. II. Effects of oral contraceptive agents. J. Clin. Endocrinol. Metab. *29*, 558—562 (1969)

25. Czernobilsky, B., Kessler, I., Lancet, M.: Cervical adenocarcinoma in a woman on long-term contraceptives. Obstet. Gynecol. *43*, 517—521 (1974)

26. Dickey, R. P., Dorr, C. H., II.: Oral contraceptives: Selection of the proper pill. Obstet. Gynecol. *33*, 273—287 (1969)

27. Dickey, R. P., Stone, S. C.: Progestational potency of oral contraceptives. Obstet. Gynecol. *47*, 106—112 (1976)

28. Diczfalusy, E.: Mode of action of contraceptive drugs. Am. J. Obstet. Gynecol. *100*, 136—163 (1968)

29. Dougherty, C. M.: Cervical cytology and sequential birth control pills. Obstet. Gynecol. *36*, 741—744 (1970)

30. Drill, V. A., Martin, D. P., Hart, E. R., McConnell, R. G.: Effects of oral contraceptives on the mammary glands of Rhesus monkeys: a preliminary report. J. Natl. Cancer Inst. *52*, 1655—1657 (1974)

31. FDA Drug Bull. *6*, 26—27 (1976)

32. Fechner, R. E.: Atypical leiomyomas and synthetic progestin therapy. Am. J. Clin. Pathol. *49*, 697—703 (1968)

33. Fechner, R. E.: Fibroadenomas in patients receiving oral contraceptives: a clinical and pathologic study. Am. J. Clin. Pathol. *53*, 857—864 (1970a)

34. Fechner, R. E.: Fibrocystic disease in women receiving oral contraceptive hormones. Cancer *25*, 1332—1339 (1970b)

35. Fechner, R. E.: The surgical pathology of the reproductive system and breast during oral contraceptive therapy. In: Genital and Mammary Pathology Decennial 1966—1975. Sommers, S. C. (Ed.). New York: Appleton-Century Crofts, 1975, pp. 103—126

36. Flowers, C. E., Jr., Vorys, N., Stevens, V., Miller, A. T., Jensen, L.: The effects of suppression of menstruation with ethynodiol diacetate upon the pituitary, ovary, and endometrium. Am. J. Obstet. Gynecol. *96*, 784—803 (1966)

37. Fredricsson, B., Bjorkman, N.: Morphologic alterations in the human oviduct epithelium induced by contraceptive steroids. Fertil. Steril. *24*, 19—30 (1973)

38. Gambrell, R. D., Jr., Bernard, D. M., Sanders, B. I., Vanderburg, N., Buxton, S. J.: Changes in sexual drives of patients on oral contraceptives. J. Reprod. Med. *17*, 165—171 (1976)

39. Gambrell, R. D., Jr., Greenblatt, R. B., Mahesh, V. B.: Postpill and pill-related amenorrhea-galactorrhea. Am. J. Obstet. Gynecol. *110*, 838—848 (1971)

40. Gershon-Cohen, J., Berger, S. M., Klickstein, H. S.: Roentgenography of breast cancer moderating concept of "biologic predeterminism". Cancer *16*, 961—964 (1963)

41. Goldenberg, V. E., Wiegenstein, L., Mottet, N. K.: Florid breast fibroadenomas in patients taking hormonal oral contraceptives. Am. J. Clin. Pathol. *49*, 52—59 (1968)

42. Golditch, I. M.: Postcontraceptive amenorrhea. Obstet. Gynecol. *39*, 903—908 (1972)

43. Goldzieher, J. W., Maqueo, M., Ricaud, L., Aguilar, J. A., Canales, E.: Induction of degenerative changes in uterine myomas by high-dosage progestin therapy. Am. J. Obstet. Gynecol. *96*, 1078—1087 (1966)

44. Gonzalez-Angulo, A., Salazar, H.: Pathology of the reproductive system, breast and liver in women during hormonal contraception. In: Uterine Contraction: Side Effects of Steroidal Contraceptives. Josimovich, J. B. (Ed.). New York: John Wiley and Sons, Inc., 1973, pp. 343—380

45. Gould, V. E., Wolff, M., Mottet, N. K.: Morphologic features of mammary carcinomas in women taking hormonal contraceptives. Am. J. Clin. Pathol. *57*, 139—143 (1972)

46. Graham, J., Graham, R., Hirabayashi, K.: Reversible "cancer" and the contraceptive pill: Report of a case. Obstet. Gynecol. *31*, 190—192 (1968)

47. Greenblatt, D. J., Koch-Weser, J.: Oral contraceptives and hypertension: A report from the Boston Collaborative Drug Surveillance Program. Obstet. Gynecol. *44*, 412—417 (1974)

48. IARC Monographs on the Evaluation of Carcinogenic Risk of Chemicals to Man: Sex Hormones. Lyon: World Health Organization, International Agency for Research on Cancer, 1974, pp. 29—30

49. Inman, W. H. W., Vessey, M. P.: Investigation of deaths from pulmonary, coronary, and cerebral thrombosis and embolism in women of child-bearing age. Br. Med. J. 2, 193–199 (1968)
50. Irey, N. S., Norris, H. J.: Intimal vascular lesions associated with female reproductive steroids. Arch. Pathol. 96, 227–234 (1973)
51. Irey, N. S., Manion, W. C., Taylor, H. B.: Vascular lesions in women taking oral contraceptives. Arch. Pathol. 89, 1–8 (1970)
52. Jackson, J. L., Spain, W. T.: Comparative study of combined and sequential antiovulatory therapy on vaginal moniliasis. Am. J. Obstet. Gynecol. 101, 1134–1135 (1968)
53. Jensen, H. K., Hansen, P. A., Blom, J.: Incidence of Candida albicans in women using oral contraceptives. Acta Obstet. Gynecol. Scand. 49, 293–296 (1970)
54. Kaufman, R. H., Reeves, K. O., Dougherty, C. M.: Severe atypical endometrial changes and sequential contraceptive use. JAMA 236, 923–926 (1976)
55. Kelley, H. W., Miles, P. A., Buster, J. E., Scragg, W. H.: Adenocarcinoma of the endometrium in women taking sequential oral contraceptives. Obstet. Gynecol. 47, 200–202 (1976)
56. Kirschstein, R. L., Rabson, A. S., Rusten, G. W.: Infiltrating duct carcinoma of the mammary gland of a Rhesus monkey after administration of an oral contraceptive. A preliminary report. J. Natl. Cancer Inst. 48, 551–556 (1972)
57. Kistner, R. W.: Endometrial alterations associated with estrogen and estrogen-progestin combinations. In: International Academy of Pathology Monograph Number 14, The Uterus. Norris, H. J., Hertig, A. T., Abell, M. R. (Eds.). Baltimore: Williams and Wilkins Co., 1973, pp. 227–254
58. Kline, T. S., Holland, M., Wemple, D.: Atypical cytology with contraceptive hormone medication. Am. J. Clin. Pathol. 53, 215–222 (1970)
59. Koide, S. S., Lyle, K. C.: Unusual signs and symptoms associated with oral contraceptive medication. J. Reprod. Med. 15, 214–224 (1975)
60. Kurman, R. J., Norris, H. J.: Adenosis. (Letter to the Editor.) Obstet. Gynecol. 46, 373–374 (1975)
61. Kusama, S., Spratt, J. S., Donegan, W. L., Watson, F. R., Cunningham, C.: The gross rates of growth of human mammary carcinoma. Cancer 30, 594–599 (1972)
62. Kyriakos, M., Kempson, R. L., Konikov, N. F.: A clinical and pathologic study of endocervical lesions associated with oral contraceptives. Cancer 22, 99–110 (1968)
63. Leis, H. P., Black, M. M., Sall, S.: The pill and the breast. J. Reprod. Med. 16, 5–9 (1976)
64. Liu, W., Koebel, L., Shipp, J., Prisby, H.: Cytologic changes following the use of oral contraceptives. Obstet. Gynecol. 30, 228–232 (1967)
65. Livingston, G. A., Joel, R. V.: The promiscuity pill principle (P-P-P). (Letter to the Editor.) Acta Cytol. 20, 4 (1976)
66. Low, J., Oparil, S.: Oral contraceptive pill hypertension. J. Reprod. Med. 15, 201–208 (1975)
67. Lyon, F. A.: The development of adenocarcinoma of the endometrium in young women receiving long-term sequential oral contraception (report of four cases). Am. J. Obstet. Gynecol. 123, 299–301 (1975)
68. Lyon, F. A., Frisch, M. J.: Endometrial abnormalities occurring in young women on long-term sequential oral contraception. Obstet. Gynecol. 47, 639–643 (1976)
69. Mahgoub, S. El, Karim, M., Ammar, R.: Long term effects of injected progestogens on the morphology of human oviducts. J. Reprod. Med. 8, 288–292 (1972)
70. Maqueo, M., Rice-Wray, E., Calderon, J. J., Goldzieher, J. W.: Ovarian morphology and prolonged use of steroid contraceptives. Contraception 5, 177–185 (1972)
71. Marshall, J. M.: The physiology of the endometrium. In: International Academy of Pathology Monograph Number 14, The Uterus. Norris, H. J., Hertig, A. T., Abell, M. R. (Eds.). Baltimore: Williams and Wilkins Co., 1973, pp. 89–109
72. Masi, A. T., Dugdale, M.: Cerebrovascular diseases associated with the use of oral contraceptives: A review of the English-language literature. Ann. Intern. Med. 72, 111–121 (1970)

73. McQuarrie, G.: Oral contraception. Med. Clin. North Am. *51*, 1261—1275 (1967)

74. Melamed, M. R., Flehinger, B. J.: Early incidence rates of precancerous cervical lesions in women using contraceptives. Gynecol. Oncol. *1*, 290—298 (1973)

75. Melamed, M. R., Koss, L. G., Flehinger, B. J., Kelisky, R. P., Dubrow, H.: Prevalence rates of uterine cervical carcinoma in situ for women using the diaphragm or contraceptive oral steroids. Br. Med. J. *3*, 195—200 (1969)

76. Moghissi, K. S.: Endometrium and endosalpinx of women treated with microdose progestogens. J. Reprod. Med. *14*, 217—218 (1975)

77. Moghissi, K. S., Syner, F. M., McBridge, L. C.: Contraceptive mechanism of microdose norethindrone. Obstet. Gynecol. *41*, 585—594 (1973)

78. Nelson, L. W., Weikel, J. H., Jr., Reno, F. E.: Mammary nodules in dogs during four years' treatment with megestrol acetate or chlormadinone acetate. J. Natl. Cancer Inst. *51*, 1303—1311 (1973)

79. Ober, W. B.: Synthetic progestagen-oestrogen preparations and endometrial morphology. J. Clin. Pathol. *19*, 138—147 (1966)

80. Ober, W. B.: Effects of oral and intrauterine contraceptives on the utrus, ovaries and other organs. Hum. Pathol. *8*, 513—517 (1977)

81. Ober, W. B., Decker, A., Clyman, M. J., Roland, M.: Endometrial morphology after sequential medication with mestranol and chlormadinone. Obstet. Gynecol. *28*, 247—253 (1966)

82. Oberti, C., Dabancens, A., Garcia-Huidobro, M., Rodriguez-Bravo, R., Zarnartu, J.: Low dosage oral progestogens to control fertility: II. Morphologic modifications in the gonad and oviduct. Obstet. Gynecol. *43*, 285—294 (1974)

83. Ory, H., Naib, Z., Conger, S. B., Hatcher, R. A., Tyler, C. W., Jr.: Contraceptive choice and prevalance of cervical dysplasia and carcinoma in situ. Am. J. Obstet. Gynecol. *124*, 573—577 (1976)

84. Osterholzer, H. O., Grillo, D., Kruger, P. S., Dunnihoo, D. R.: The effect of oral contraceptive steroids on branches of the uterine artery. Obstet. Gynecol. *49*, 227—232 (1977)

85. Patek, E., Nilsson, L., Johannisson, E., Hellema, M., Bout, J.: Scanning electron microscopic study of the human fallopian tube. Report III. The effect of midpregnancy and of various steroids. Fertil. Steril. *24*, 31—43 (1973)

86. Pearlman, A. W.: Breast cancer — influence of growth rate on prognosis and treatment evaluation. A study based on mastectomy scar recurrences. Cancer *38*, 1826—1833 (1976)

87. Penman, H. G.: The effect of oral contraceptives on the histology of carcinoma of the breast. J. Pathol. *101*, 66—68 (1970)

88. Phillips, N., Duffy, T.: One-hour glucose tolerance in relation to the use of contraceptive drugs. Am. J. Obstet. Gynecol. *116*, 91—100 (1973)

89. Piiroinen, O., Rauramo, L.: Oral contraception and uterine size — ultrasonic study. Am. J. Obstet. Gynecol. *122*, 349—351 (1975)

90. Plate, W. P.: Ovarian changes after long term oral contraception. Acta Endocrinol. *55*, 71—77 (1967)

91. Posner, N. A., Silverstone, F. A., Tobin, E. H., Breuer, J.: Changes in carbohydrate tolerance during longterm oral contraception. Am. J. Obstet. Gynecol. *123*, 119—127 (1975)

92. Prakash, S., Scully, R. E.: Sarcoma-like pseudopregnancy changes in uterine leiomyomas: report of a case resulting from prolonged norethindrone therapy. Obstet. Gynecol. *24*, 106—109 (1964)

93. Reynolds, S. R. M.: In: Physiology of the Uterus. 2nd ed. New York: Hafner Publishing Company, 1965, Ch. 14, pp. 194—202

94. Rice-Wray, E., Carreu, S., Gorodovsky, J., Esquivel, J., Goldzieher, J. W.: Return of ovulation after discontinuance of oral contraceptives. Fertil. Steril. *18*, 212—218 (1967)

95. Robboy, S. J., Welch, W. R.: Microglandular hyperplasia in vaginal adenosis associated with oral contraceptives and prenatal diethylstilbestrol exposure. Obstet. Gynecol. *49*, 430—434 (1977)

96. Robson, J. S., Martin, A. M., Ruckley, V. A., MacDonald, M. K.: Irreversible post-partum renal failure: A new syndrome. Q. J. Med. *37*, 423—435 (1968)

97. Roland, M., Clyman, M. J., Decker, A., Ober, W. B.: Classification of endometrial response to synthetic progestogen-estrogen compounds. Fertil. Steril. *15*, 143—163 (1964)

98. Roland, M., Clyman, M. J., Decker, A., Ober, W. B.: Sequential endometrial alterations during one cycle of treatment with synthetic progestagen-estrogen compounds. Fertil. Steril. *17*, 338—350 (1966)

99. Ryan, G. M., Jr., Craig, J., Reid, D. E.: Histology of the uterus and ovaries after long-term cyclic norethynodrel therapy. Am. J. Obstet. Gynecol. *90*, 715—725 (1964)

100. Sandmire, H. F., Austin, S. D., Bechtel, R. C.: Carcinoma of the cervix in oral contraceptive steroid and IUD users and nonusers. Am. J. Obstet. Gynecol. *125*, 339—345 (1976)

101. Sartwell, P. E., Arthes, F. G., Tonascia, J. A.: Epidemiology of benign breast lesions: Lack of association with oral contraceptive use. New. Engl. J. Med *288*, 551—554 (1973)

102. Sartwell, P. E., Masi, A. T., Arthes, F. G., Greene, G. R., Smith, H. E.: Thromboembolism and oral contraceptives: an epidemiologic case-control study. Am. J. Epidemiol. *90*, 365—380 (1969)

103. Second report on the oral contraceptives, Advisory Committee on Obstetrics and Gynecology, Food and Drug Administration, Washington, D.C.: U.S. Government Printing Office, 1969

104. Shulman, J. J., Merritt, C. G.: Contraceptive choice and cervical cytology. Am. J. Obstet. Gynecol. *116*, 1079—1087 (1973)

105. Silverberg, S. G., Makowski, E. L.: Endometrial carcinoma in young women taking oral contraceptive agents. Obstet. Gynecol. *46*, 503—506 (1975)

106. Silverberg, S. G., Makowski, E. L., Roche, W. D.: Endometrial carcinoma in women under 40 years of age. Comparison of cases in oral contraceptive users and non-users. Cancer *39*, 592—598 (1977)

107. Smith, R. W.: Hypertension and oral contraception. Am. J. Obstet. Gynecol. *113*, 482—487 (1972)

108. Song, J., Mark, M. S., Lawler, M. P., Jr.: Endometrial changes in women receiving oral contraceptives. Am. J. Obstet. Gynecol. *107*, 717—728 (1970)

109. Spellacy, W. N.: A review of carbohydrate metabolism and the oral contraceptives. Am. J. Obstet. Gynecol. *104*, 448—460 (1969)

110. Spellacy, W. N.: Progestogen and estrogen effects on carbohydrate metabolism. In: Uterine Contraction — Side Effects of Steroidal Contraceptives. Josimovich, J. B. (Ed.). New York: John Wiley & Sons, Inc., 1973, pp. 327—341

111. Spellacy, W. N.: Metabolic effects of oral contraceptives. Clin. Obstet. Gynecol. *17*, 53—64 (1974)

112. Spellacy, W. N., Buhi, W. C., Birk, S. A., McCreary, S. A.: Change in glucose and insulin after six months treatment with the oral contraceptive Demulen. Am. J. Obstet. Gynecol. *119*, 266—267 (1974)

113. Spellacy, W. N., Zaias, N., Buhi, W. C., Birk, S. A.: Vaginal yeast growth and contraceptive practices. Obstet. Gynecol. *38*, 343—349 (1971)

114. Speroff, L., Glass, R. H., Kase, N. G.: Clinical Gynecologic Endocrinology and Infertility. Baltimore: The Williams and Wilkins Company, 1973, pp. 101—102

115. Speroff, L., Glass, R. H., Kase, N. G.: Clinical Gynecologic Endocrinology and Infertility. Baltimore: The Williams and Wilkins Company, 1973, pp. 152—171

116. Steele, S. J., Mason, B., Brett, A.: Amenorrhea after discontinuing combined oestrogen-progestogen oral contraceptives. Br. Med. J. *4*, 343—345 (1973)

117. Stern, E., Forsythe, A. B., Youkeles, L., Coffelt, C. F.: Steroid contraceptive use and cervical dysplasia: increased risk of progression. Science *196*, 1460—1462 (1977)

118. Taber, B. F.: Breast cancer and oral contraception. J. Reprod. Med. *15*, 97—99 (1975)

119. Tapia, H. R., Johnson, C. E., Strong, C. G.: Effect of oral contraceptive therapy on the renin-angiotension system in normotensive and hypertensive women. Obstet. Gynecol. *41*, 643–649 (1973)

120. Taylor, H. B.: Oral contraceptives and pathologic changes in the breast. Cancer *28*, 1388–1390 (1971)

121. Taylor, H. B., Irey, N. S., Norris, H. J.: Atypical endocervical hyperplasia in women taking oral contraceptives. JAMA *202*, 637–639 (1967)

122. Tobon, H.: Malignant hypertension, uremia and hemolytic anemia in a patient on oral contraceptives. Obstet. Gynecol. *40*, 681–685 (1972)

123. Tyson, J. E., Andreasson, B., Huth, J., Smith, B., Zacur, H.: Neuroendocrine dysfunction in galactorrhea — amenorrhea after oral contraceptive use. Obstet. Gynecol. *46*, 1–11 (1975)

124. Vessey, M. P.: Thromboembolism, cancer and oral contraceptives. Clin. Obstet. Gynecol. *17*, 65–78 (1974)

125. Vessey, M. P., Doll, R.: Investigation of relation between use of oral contraceptives and thromboembolic disease. Br. Med. J. *2*, 199–205 (1968)

126. Vessey, M. P., Doll, R., Sutton, P. M.: Investigation of the possible relationship between oral contraceptives and benign and malignant breast disease. Cancer *28*, 1395–1399 (1971)

127. Vessey, M. P., Doll, R., Sutton, P. M.: Oral contraceptives and breast neoplasia: A retrospective study. Br. Med. J. *3*, 719–724 (1972)

128. Wagoner, R. D., Holley, K. E., Johnson, W. J.: Accelerated nephrosclerosis and postpartum acute renal failure in normotensive patients. Ann. Intern. Med. *69*, 237–248 (1968)

129. Wiegenstein, L., Tank, R., Gould, V. E.: Multiple breast fibroadenomas in women on hormonal contraceptives. (Letter to the Editor.) New. Engl. J. Med. *284*, 676 (1971)

130. Wilkinson, E., Dufour, D. R.: Pathogenesis of microglandular hyperplasia of the cervix uteri. Obstet. Gynecol. *47*, 189–195 (1976)

131. Wright, S. W., Fotherby, K., Fairweather, F.: Effect of daily small doses of Norgestrel on ovarian function. J. Obstet. Gynecol. *77*, 65–68 (1970)

132. Zacharle, B. J., Richardson, J. A.: Irreversible renal failure secondary to hypertension induced by oral contraceptives. Ann. Intern. Med. *77*, 83–85 (1972)

133. Zussman, W. V., Forbes, D. A., Carpenter, R. J.: Ovarian morphology following cyclic norethindrone — mestranol therapy. Am. J. Obstet. Gynecol. *99*, 99–105 (1967)

Hepatic Neoplasms Associated with Contraceptive and Anabolic Steroids[1]

Kamal G. Ishak

An association between hepatocellular adenoma (HCA) and oral contraceptives (OC) was first pointed out by BAUM et al. in 1973 [12]. Other examples followed as well as reports of possible associations between OC and focal nodular hyperplasia (FNH), hepatocellular carcinoma (HCC), and other malignant hepatic tumors [1, 3–5, 7–10, 17, 20, 21, 23, 24, 26–28, 31, 32, 35, 43, 44, 49, 51–56, 59, 65, 71, 74, 77, 80, 84, 90, 92–95, 100–102, 105, 111, 115, 116, 120, 126, 129, 133, 137, 141, 143–145, 147, 148]. The occurrence of HCC and other tumors of the liver in patients receiving anabolic steroids has been the subject of many reports [18, 22, 48, 57, 61, 64, 72, 73, 78, 86, 99, 103, 108, 119, 121, 127, 128, 139, 155]. Likewise a number of editorials [37–40, 134] and several reviews have dealt with tumors of the liver associated with OC [49, 79, 114, 123, 131].

The confusion in the literature between the entities of HCA and FNH is indeed unfortunate since it is highly probable that FNH is not etiologically related to the use of OC whereas HCA is. This state of affairs has also made it very difficult to deal with the flood of reported cases that followed the study of BAUM et al. [12] and has been made even worse by review articles reclassifying the pathology of the published tumors.

The purpose of this presentation is to emphasize the differences between HCA and FNH and to examine the current state of knowledge regarding their association with OC. The occasional occurrence of nodular regenerative hyperplasia (NRH) in patients on OC or anabolic steroids (AS) is discussed in the light of other nonsteroid associated cases. Malignant tumors of the liver that have been reported in patients using OC or AS will also be reviewed.

Focal Nodular Hyperplasia

A benign tumor of the liver has also been referred to as focal cirrhosis, hepatic pseudotumor, solitary hyperplastic nodule, hemartomatous cholangiohepatoma, hepatic hamartoma, and mixed adenoma. Unfortunately the terms adenoma and benign hepatoma have also occasionally been used for FNH. The most widely used term, FNH, was first introduced by EDMONDSON [42] in 1958 and is the one adopted by the World Health Organization in 1975 [154] and by the Fogarty International Center and the International Association for the Study of the Liver in 1976 [85].

Although FNH occurs in both sexes and at all ages, many more cases occur in females and more of the reported tumors have been described in adults. The experience of the author with

---

1 The opinions and assertions contained herein are the private views of the authors and are not to be construed as official or as reflecting the views of the Department of the Army or the Department of Defense.

ten cases of FNH occurring in the pediatric age group together with a review of the literature was recently published [69]. With reference to the sex incidence, FNH is at least twice as frequent in females as in males; in a series of 130 patients studied by the author there were 86 females and 44 males [70]. Only 20% of the patients with FNH had symptoms and signs related to their neoplasm; in the remainder the FNH was discovered incidentally at surgery (58 patients), usually for diseases of the gallbladder, or at necropsy (46 patients). The majority (15 of 20) of the patients with symptoms and signs had a mass either discovered by the patient or palpated during a routine physical checkup. Pain or discomfort was associated with the mass in five patients; the mass in one of these patients was tender and pulsatile and a loud bruit was heard over it. Two of the patients with negative physical findings had symptoms mimicking those of peptic ulcer or cholelithiasis; in both patients subsequent laparotomy revealed pressure of the FNH on the stomach and gallbladder, respectively. Another patient experienced pain on pressure over the FNH, although no mass was palpated. One female had an acute abdominal crisis due to rupture of her FNH. Three patients had manifestations of portal hypertension associated with multiple FNH. One of the patients with portal hypertension, an 8-year-old child, had left hemihypertrophy; this patient was reported by EVERSON et al. [46].

The majority of patients with FNH have normal results of tests of hepatic function. The tumor(s) will generally show up as a filling defect(s) by hepatic scan. Indentation of and pressure on adjacent hollow viscera may be demonstrated by upper and lower gastrointestinal radiographic studies, intravenous pyelography, and cholecystography [69]. Angiographic studies of FNH have been reported by GOLDSTEIN et al. [55], HOLDER et al. [64], McLOUGH-LIN et al. [98], and McLOUGHLIN and GILDAY [97], and FECHNER and ROEHM [50]. According to FECHNER and ROEHM [50], when FNH is visualized arteriographically an artery enters the lesion, branches, and supplies the mass centrifugally. It is likely that the central fibrous zone is the area from which these branches originate. These authors are of the opinion that these features contrast with arteriograms of HCA in which the blood flow is centripetal. In HCA numerous small feeding arteries surround the sharply marginated tumor and send many small vessels into the mass.

The location of FNH in the liver in the 130 cases studied by the author is shown in Table 1. Of these patients 78.5% had a single tumor mass, 12.3% had two nodules, 6.9% had multiple nodules, and 2.3% had left lobar nodular hyperplasia. The uncommon lobar distribution of FNH is reported in only one other patient [142]. The majority of patients (84.0%) had a single

Table 1. Focal nodular hyperplasia. Location of nodules in liver

Type of lesion	Number of cases	Distribution					
		Right lobe	Left lobe	Both lobes	Caudate lobe	Riedel's lobe	Unknown
Single nodule	102	59	32	—	3	1	7
Two nodules	16	3	4	8	—	—	1
Multiple nodules	9	1	1	7	—	—	—
Lobar	3	—	3	—	—	—	—
Total	130	63	40	15	3	1	8

nodule measuring 5 cm or less in diameter. In sixteen patients (12.7%) the FNH measured 5—10 cm in diameter, while in four patients (3.2%) the FNH had a diameter greater than 10 cm.

The gross appearance of FNH is highly characteristic. The lesions are usually globular, lobulated, and often partly project from one of the surfaces of the liver. Only a few (4.6%) of the tumors have a pedicle. Prominent vessels are often seen coursing over the surface. The consistency is firm to rubbery and when transected the tumor often bulges above the plane of the rest of the liver (Fig. 1). Focal nodular hyperplasia is usually wellcircumscribed but nonencapsulated. The color is invariably lighter than that of the adjacent parenchyma and varies from light brown to tan to yellow. Areas of hemorrhage, necrosis or infarction are not seen. The pathognomonic gross feature of FNH is its subdivision into smaller nodules by fibrous septa that often run into retracted stellate scars; the latter may be central or eccentric and, particularly in larger lesions, there may be several of them (Fig. 1). FNH is not associated with cirrhosis or other intrinsic diseases of the liver.

In 3 of the 130 cases from the Armed Forces Institute of Pathology (AFIP) cavernous hemangiomas (single in two cases and multiple in one) were found in the same liver harboring the FNH. A much higher association with hemangiomas (20.6%) was reported in the autopsy series of FNH published by BENZ and BAGGENSTOSS [16]. A number of the patients with FNH had benign or malignant neoplasms of other organs, but not all of them were found simultaneously with the discovery of the FNH. Occasionally patients with FNH may also have HCA (See section on HCA). One interesting association is glioblastoma multiforme, which was found in four of the AFIP patients and was also reported in another patient [45]. Diseases of the gallbladder are, in the author's experience, frequently associated with FNH. Forty (30.8%) of the patients had cholelithiasis and/or chronic cholecystitis or cholesterolosis; thirty-three of the patients were female.

Microscopic examination of FNH usually reveals a tumor that is sharply circumscribed from the adjacent, often compressed hepatic parenchyma (Fig. 2). The epithelial component of the

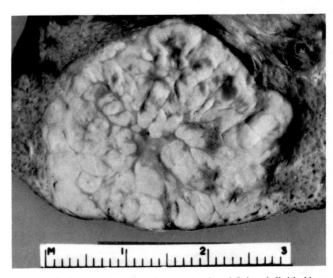

Fig. 1. Cut sections of FNH. The lesion is well circumscribed but nonencapsulated. It is subdivided into small nodules by fibrous septa. Note the *central* retracted scar

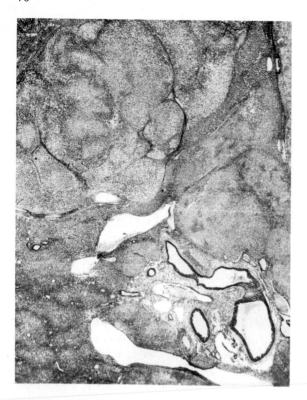

Fig. 2. Focal nodular hyperplasia (*upper two-thirds* of photomicrograph) is divided into subunits by fibrous septa. A portal area with large arteries and veins (*lower third* of photomicrograph) is interposed between the FNH and the adjacent parenchyma. AFIP Neg. No. 74-3864, Masson's trichrome, × 9

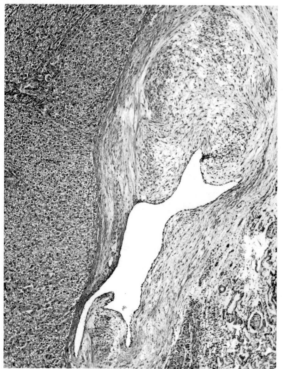

Fig. 3. Vein in FNH shows eccentric thickening of the wall due to fibromuscular hyperplasia. AFIP Neg. No. 75-5136, Masson's trichrome, × 70

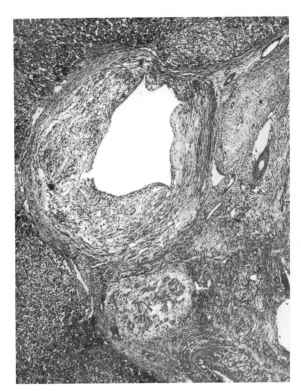

Fig. 4. Concentric subintimal fibrosis of vein in FNH. AFIP Neg. No. 75-6303, Masson's trichrome, × 70

neoplasm is divided into smaller units by the fibrous septa that may be linked to the stellate scars. The vasculature consists of arteries, veins, and sinusoids. The largest vessels are seen at the junction of the FNH with the adjacent parenchyma and in the stellate scars. These vessels, regardless of the sex or age of the patient, characteristically show eccentric or concentric thickening due to fibromuscular hyperplasia (Figs. 3—5). The change most frequently involves veins (Figs. 3 and 4), but arteries are also occasionally affected; when this happens the elastica may show fragmentation or reduplication (Fig. 5). The author agrees with FECHNER and ROEHM [50] that the vascular changes in FNH resemble those seen in arteriovenous malformations at other sites. In addition to vessels, medium and large bile ducts and nerve fibers are often found at the periphery of FNH.

A very characteristic histologic feature of FNH is the presence of small bile ducts in the septa, particularly at the interface with the parenchyma, which are supported by a basement membrane (Figs. 6 and 7). The ducts may be surrounded by and infiltrated with neutrophils. Mucin production by the lining cells is not demonstrable by special stains, such as the mucicarmine stain. Variable numbers of inflammatory cells, predominantly lymphocytes, may be found infiltrating the fibrous septa (Figs. 8 and 9).

The epithelial component of FNH consists of cells resembling normal hepatocytes arranged in plates that are two-cells thick (Figs. 10 and 11). There is no normal lobular architecture. The sinusoids between the plates are inconspicuous and are lined by flat endothelial cells, which generally show no evidence of phagocytic activity. A reticulum framework is always demonstrable in silver preparations (Fig.12).

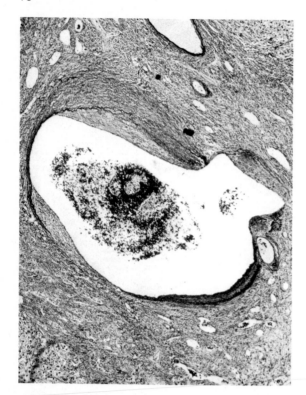

Fig. 5. Artery in FNH shows eccentric subintimal fibrosis. Note disruption and reduplication of the internal elastic lamina. AFIP Neg. No. 69—7703, Movat's pentachrome, × 60

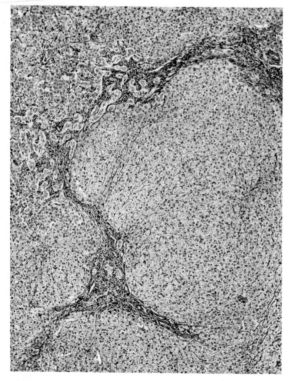

Fig. 6. Septum in FNH is moderately infiltrated with inflammatory cells and contains many small ducts. The epithelial component shows no lobular architecture. AFIP Neg. No. 75-6301, H & E × 60

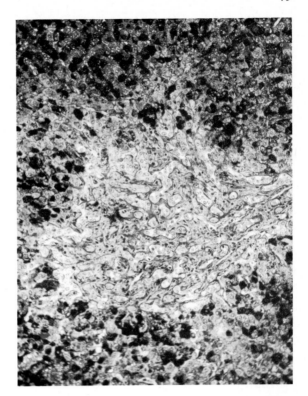

Fig. 7. Transversely sectioned septum in FNH shows numerous small bile ducts. Cells in surrounding epithelial component are darkly stained because of the large quantity of glycogen in their cytoplasm. AFIP Neg. No. 74-5155, PAS, × 165

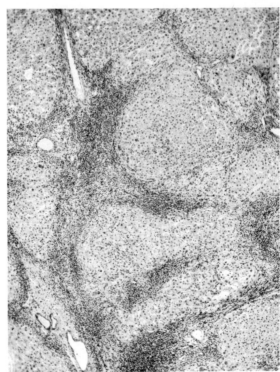

Fig. 8. Septa of FNH are heavily infiltrated with inflammatory cells. AFIP Neg. No. 64-5583, H & E, × 50

80 Kamal G. Ishak

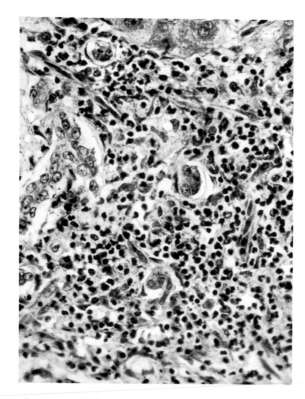

Fig. 9. Most of inflammatory cells in septum of this FNH are lymphocytes. AFIP Neg. No. 74-5152, H & E, × 440

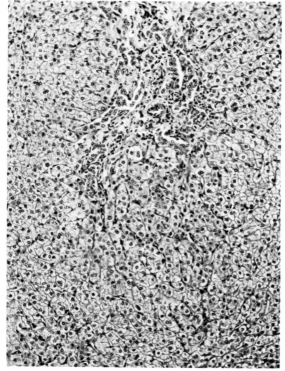

Fig. 10. Cells of the epithelial component of FNH show little variation in size and the majority contain one nucleus. AFIP Neg. No. 75-5146, H & E, × 130

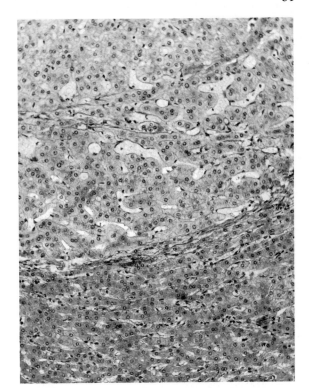

Fig. 11. Cells of FNH (*top two-thirds* of photomicrograph) are larger and paler than those of adjacent parenchyma. Cells are arranged in plates that are two-cells thick. Nuclei are approximately equal in size to those of the normal hepatocytes. AFIP Neg. No. 76-10510, H & E, × 145

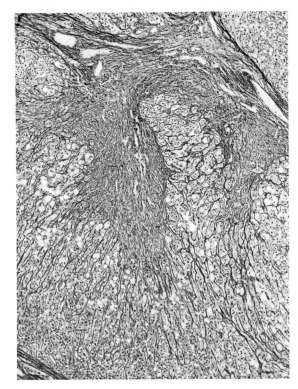

Fig. 12. The septa of this FNH contain numerous reticulum fibers and the cells of the epithelial component are supported by a well-developed reticulum framework. AFIP Neg. No. 74–3871, Manuel's reticulum, × 50

Bile canaliculi are present between the cells but are not dilated. The cells show moderate variation in size and have well-defined cell membranes. The cytoplasm is eosinophilic but may be vacuolated due to the presence of fat. The majority of the tumors contain fat (demonstrable by an oil-red 0 stain of frozen sections) and glycogen; the latter is usually in excess of that in the adjacent parenchyma (Figs. 7, 13, and 14). Globular inclusions (PAS-positive or negative) or Mallory's bodies are not seen in the cytoplasm. Rarely FNH may show a few ballooned hepatocytes or a sinusoidal acidophilic body at the junction of the epithelial component with the septa (Figs. 15 and 16). Lipofuscin pigment is generally not demonstrable in the cells of FNH (Fig. 17) and the stains for hemosiderin are negative. Occasionally tumors may contain a small quantity of copper. Most of the cells have a single, centrally placed nucleus, which is about the same size as that of hepatocytes in the adjacent parenchyma (Fig. 11). The nuclei are normochromatic and have small nucleoli; no mitoses are seen. No bile is found in the cytoplasm or canaliculi of the cells in the majority of cases. The tumor cells are, however, capable of producing bile since cholestasis may be present in FNH (as well as the rest of the liver) in the occasional patient who also has extrahepatic obstruction; two such cases are on file at AFIP.

An ultrastructural study of FNH by PHILLIPS et al. [117] has shown that the hepatocytes are cytologically normal but contain excess glycogen. In contrast to the normal liver FNH shows anomalous microvilli on the plasma membranes of contiguous hepatocytes.

FNH arises in a liver that usually shows no significant pathology. Depending on the size of the tumor there may be some compression strophy of the immediately adjacent parenchyma. Some lesions of the nonneoplastic liver, e.g., cholestasis in extrahepatic biliary obstruction,

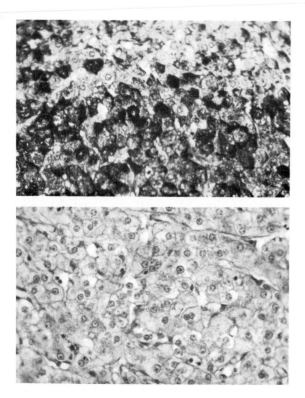

Fig. 13. Glycogen in cells of FNH (*top half* of field) is removed by predigestion with diastase. AFIP Neg. No. 74-5154, PAS before and after diastase digestion, × 300

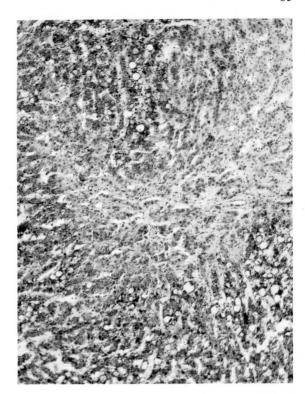

Fig. 14. Cells of FNH contain a moderate quantity of neutral lipid in the form of fine vacuoles. AFIP Neg. No. 74-3873, Frozen section with oil-red 0, × 75

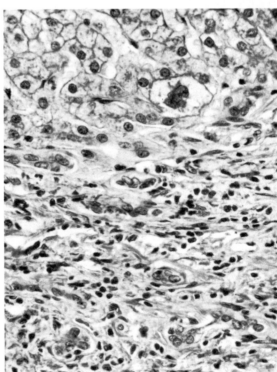

Fig. 15. Ballooned cell of FNH adjacent to a fibrous septum. AFIP Neg. No. 73-9540, H & E, × 395

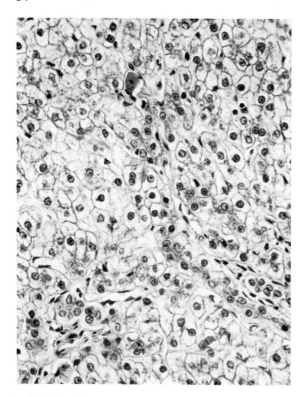

Fig. 16. Sinusoidal acidophilic body in FNH. Note uniformity of cells, empty or lightly stained cytoplasm, and the small nuclei. AFIP Neg. No. 73-9539, H & E, × 300

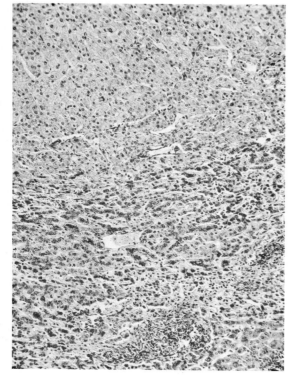

Fig. 17. Cells of the epithelial component of FNH (*upper third* of field) do not contain lipofuscin pigment whereas the adjacent parenchymal cells do. AFIP Neg. No. 76-5456, Fontana, × 100

may be reflected in the FNH, but others, e.g., severe congestion in patients with congestive heart failure, may not.

The etiology and pathogenesis of FNH have not yet been determined. A number of theories have been propounded, including a hamartomatous malformation, or a reparative process in an area of focal injury, possibly predetermined by an underlying vascular anomaly [14, 16, 42, 50, 151]. It is remarkable that there is no animal model for FNH.

The evidence against an etiologic relationship between FNH and OC has been cited by a number of authors [49, 69, 81]. Briefly, this includes the frequent finding of FNH in infants and children, in males as well as in females, and its occurrence in many females prior to the introduction of OC into clinical practice [70]. The author has seen only one case of FNH present with rupture and hemoperitoneum, a complication frequently occurring in HCA. In a recent review of the literature FECHNER [49] found that of the nine women with FNH known to be taking OC two presented with intrahepatic or intraperitoneal bleeding. He suggested that this complication could be a direct consequence of OC therapy and could occur even if the underlying lesion itself were not caused by hormone therapy. It is also conceivable that FNH, a very slowly growing neoplasm, could undergo accelerated growth under the influence of contraceptive steroids or conjugated estrogens. Such a possibility is supported by the occasional report of "regression" of FNH after discontinuation of OC or estrogen therapy [1, 126]. It is also of interest that rapid enlargement of another liver tumor, cavernous hemangioma, has been reported in a 57-year-old woman who had received an estrogen preparation for 18 months [104].

The treatment of choice of FNH is simple excision. In cases in which resection is contraindicated hepatic artery ligation may be worth a trial; the successful treatment of FNH in a 3-year-old child by this method was recently reported by MOWAT et al. [107].

The author has not seen any case of malignant transformation of FNH. There is one report of a 21-year-old female who had a HCC that was thought to have arisen in a FNH; that patient had been using OC for 2 years [35]. POPPER (cited by KLATSKIN [79]), who reviewed the sections from that tumor, is of the opinion that it was an HCA rather than a FNH. More recently, CHRISTOPHERSON et al. [28] have reported an HCC arising in a FNH.

Hepatocellular Adenoma

Although hepatocellular adenoma occurs less frequently than other benign tumors of the liver, such as FNH and cavernous hemangioma, there has been a marked increase in its incidence (based on published reports and the author's experience) since 1960 and even more so since 1970. Few cases were published from large medical centers prior to 1960 [42, 62, 91]. In an epidemiologic survey of 105 cases on file at AFIP [125] 94 of the cases (90.4%) were diagnosed between 1965 and 1976.

The data presented here are based on a study of 105 cases on file at AFIP [125]; these include the 75 cases previously published by ISHAK and RABIN [70]. All patients were women between the ages of 16 and 61, although the majority were between the third and fourth decades of life.

Almost one-third of the AFIP patients presented with an acute abdominal crisis, either due to rupture of the tumor with hemoperitoneum (22.7%) or to sudden hemorrhage and/or infarction within the tumor (9.4%). The association between rupture of HCA and menstruation that was reported by EDMONDSON et al. [43] has not been substantiated in the series studied at AFIP [125]. Two-thirds of the AFIP patients had an upper abdominal mass, with or without associated symptoms (e.g., abdominal discomfort or episodic pain, nausea, and anorexia). An unusual acute illness manifested by fever, chills, sweats, and diarrhea, and prostration with severe metabolic acidosis was reported by MINOW et al. [101] in a 22-year-old female with HCA; all symptoms resolved after resection of the tumor. Less than 10% of the AFIP patients had no symptoms or signs related to their adenoma [70]. In the majority of patients tests of hepatic function were normal; minimal to moderate elevations of transaminases and alkaline phosphatase values occurred in patients who bled into their tumor or intraperitoneally. Serum α-fetoprotein values were usually not elevated [70], a finding also reported in other cases [2, 79]. The negative α-fetoprotein determination and the absence of an additional 5' nucleotide phosphodiesterase isoenzyme in the serum [146] could be helpful in the differentiation of HCA from HCC.

Radiographic studies may show displacement of various hollow viscera and organs by the adenoma [70]. Hepatic scans often show single or multiple defects, but tumors less than 4 cm in diameter usually escape detection [79]. Angiography is perhaps the best method currently available for diagnosis [55, 71, 97, 98], although differentiation of HCA from FNH by this technique may not be possible [55]. In the review of KLATSKIN [79] 90% of cases of benign hepatic tumors associated with OC had demonstrable angiographic abnormalities. The principal features included enlargement of the hepatic artery (33%), a peripheral arterial blood supply (43%), increased vascularity (78%), and a tumor "blush" during the venous phase (38%). Whole body computer tomography has recently been utilized in diagnosis of a HCA in a patient who had taken OC for 7 years [59].

The location and distribution of HCA in 75 previously published cases [70] are shown in Table 2. Of these patients 71% had a single tumor, 13% had two tumors, and 16% had multiple tumors. Most of the tumors (66.7%) were found in the right lobe, 20.8% were in the left lobe, while 12.5% were located in both lobes of the liver.

The gross appearance of HCA is variable but clearly distinguishable from that of FNH. All of the tumors arise in noncirrhotic livers. They are usually sharply demarcated from the adjacent parenchyma; slightly more than a third (33.7%) are encapsulated (Figs. 18 and 19). A fifth of the tumors are pedunculated. Prominent vessels are usually noticeable on the external surface. The tumors are usually globular in shape and their consistency is more often soft than firm. Cut sections show a tumor(s) that is flush with the rest of the adjacent liver (Fig. 19); it may be faintly lobulated, but the stellate scars and radiating septa seen in FNH are absent. The color varies from yellow to tan to light brown; some tumors may have a green color in focal areas or at the periphery. Hemorrhages of varying size are present in the majority

Table 2. Hepatocellular adenoma. Location of tumors in liver

Type of lesion	Number of cases	Distribution			
		Right lobe	Left lobe	Both	Unknown
Single tumor	53	39	11	–	3
Two tumors	10	3	4	3	–
Multiple tumors	12	6	–	6	–
Total	75	48	15	9	3

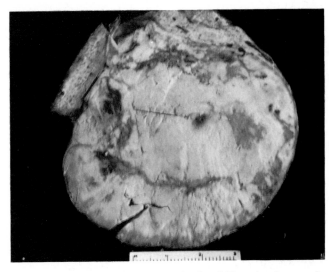

Fig. 18. Cut section of HCA. The tumor is well demarcated but nonencapsulated. Note the absence of a "substructure" and the scattered hemorrhages. AFIP Neg. No. 66-13108

(72.0%) (Fig. 18). Other gross findings include cystic or 'gelatinous' foci (7.6%), infarcts (6.0%) (Fig. 19), and foci of 'necrosis' (32.0%). The gross features of HCA are compared and contrasted with those of FNH and HCC in Table 3.

HCA may or may not be encapsulated microscopically. The vascular supply is scattered throughout the tumor, veins being more conspicuous and apparently more numerous than arteries. The largest vessels are seen at or near the surface of the tumor (Fig. 20). In the adenomas removed from patients on OC the surface vessels, particularly the arteries, frequently show intimal lesions (Figs. 21 and 22) similar to those described in other organs

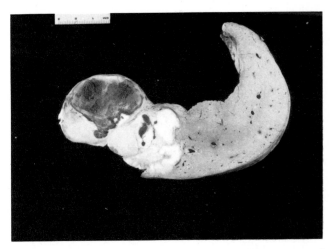

Fig. 19. Cut section of lobectomy specimen showing a sharply circumscribed HCA. Note area of infarction to the *left*. AFIP Neg. No. 70-4850

Table 3. Comparison of gross features of FNH, HCA, and HCC

Morphologic criterion	FNH	HCA	HCC
Number of nodules	Usually single	Usually single	Single or multiple
Pedicle	Rarely present	Rarely present	Absent
Surface vessels	Prominent	Prominent	Prominent or inconspicuous
Consistency	Firm to rubbery	Soft and fleshy	Soft and fleshy
Capsule	Absent	Absent or partial	Absent
Satellite nodules	Absent	Present, rare	Present
Cut surface	Subdivided into smaller units by fibrous septa	Not subdivided	Not subdivided[a]
Color	Uniform tan or yellow	Uniform or variegated brown to tan to yellow	Uniform or variegated tan to yellow to brown to green
Hemorrhages and areas of infarction	Absent	Present, frequent	Present, frequent
Cystic gelatinous degeneration	Absent	Present, rare	Absent
Adjacent liver	Noncirrhotic	Noncirrhotic	Frequently cirrhotic[a]
Invasion of vessels (e.g., portal vein), bile ducts, adjacent viscera, and organs	Absent	Absent	Present

[a] Except in cases associated with anabolic steroids.

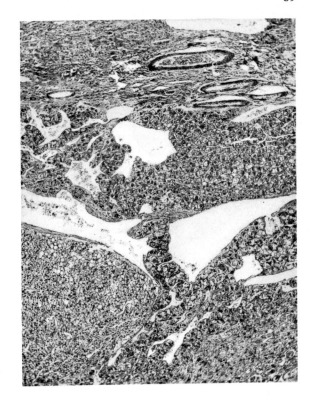

Fig. 20. Peripheral part of HCA showing large veins and several small arteries at the *top right hand corner* of thre field. AFIP Neg. No. 75-6161, H & E, × 50

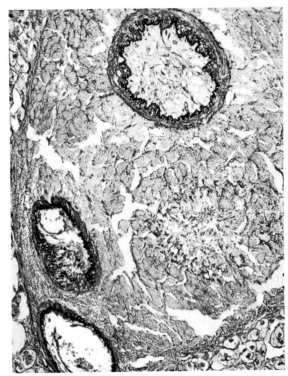

Fig. 21. Two arteries in portal area outside an HCA. They show subintimal fibrosis that, in the *top* vessel, completely occludes the lumen. AFIP Neg. No. 76-10039, Movat's pentachrome, × 165

90   Kamal G. Ishak

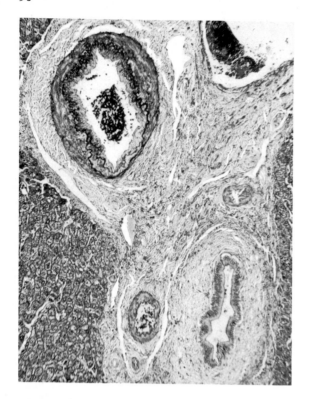

Fig. 22. Artery in portal area
adjacent to HCA showing
concentric fibrous thickening and
reduplication of the internal elastic
lamina. AFIP Neg. No. 76-10335,
Movat's pentachrome, × 90

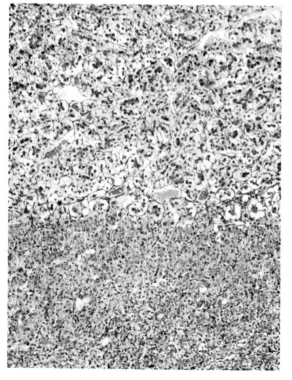

Fig. 23. HCA (*top half*) is sharply
demarcated from the adjacent
parenchyma but no capsule is
present. The cells of HCA appear
to be growing in a continuous sheet
and are larger and lighter in color
than the normal hepatocytes. AFIP
Neg. No. 73-9505, H & E, × 90

and tissues of women taking OC [67, 68, 113]. These changes are also described by HILLIARD and NORRIS in this monograph. Other than the vessels, an occasional small or medium-sized bile duct may be present at the junction of the HCA and the adjacent parenchyma (Fig. 22).

The cells of HCA are arranged in plates that are generally two-cells thick. Slitlike sinusoidal spaces, lined by flattened endothelial cells, are present between the plates. The thin plates and lack of distinctly dilated sinusoids give HCA its characteristic "sheetlike" growth pattern, an important histologic feature that distinguishes it from hepatocellular carcinoma (Figs. 23 and 24). A reticulin framework is generally lacking in HCA, except for the periphery of some tumors. In addition to the formed elements of the blood occasional tumors may contain hematopoietic cells [such as megakaryocytes (Fig. 25), erythroblasts, and nucleated erythrocytes] in the sinusoids, a finding noted by others [137].

Definite canaliculi are present between the neoplastic cells in the plates. If these are dilated the surrounding cells are arranged in a ring (pseudoglandular or pseudoacinar pattern). The dilatation is usually accompanied by the accumulation of bile in the lumen (Figs. 24 and 26). When the pseudoglandular pattern and cholestasis are conspicuous, it is the periphery of the tumor that is generally affected (Fig. 24), a feature that may also be grossly obvious.

The neoplastic cells of HCA are usually larger than hepatocytes in the nonneoplastic parenchyma (Figs. 23, 24, 27, and 28). The cell membranes are clearly defined. Most of the cells are lighter in color than normal hepatocytes and may contain small or medium-sized vacuoles (Fig. 27). The pallor of the cytoplasm is due to the large quantity of glycogen (Fig. 29), while the vacuoles represent accumulated lipid (Fig. 30); both glycogen and fat are

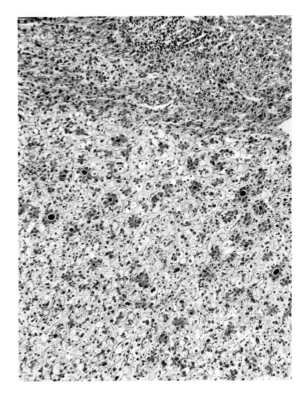

Fig. 24. Superficial part of HCA has similar features to those noted in Figure 23 but also shows multiple bile-filled pseudoglands. AFIP Neg. No. 76-10034, H & E, × 90

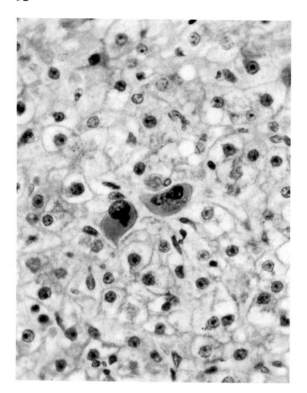

Fig. 25. Sinusoid in HCA contains two megakaryocytes. AFIP Neg. No. 68-2203, H & E, × 530

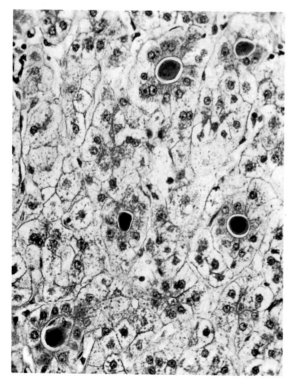

Fig. 26. Several pseudoglands contain bile plugs in the lumen. AFIP Neg. No. 76-10047, H & E, × 300

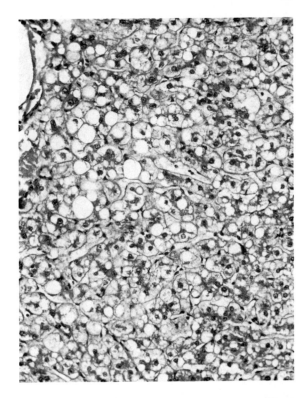

Fig. 27. Cells of HCA show uniformity of size and have a pale cytoplasm containing varying-sized lipid vacuoles. AFIP Neg. No. 73-8842, H & E, × 180

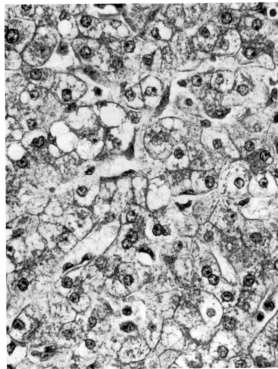

Fig. 28. Nuclei of cells of HCA occupy a relatively small part of the cell volume and have inconspicuous nucleoli. AFIP Neg. No. 74-5458, H & E

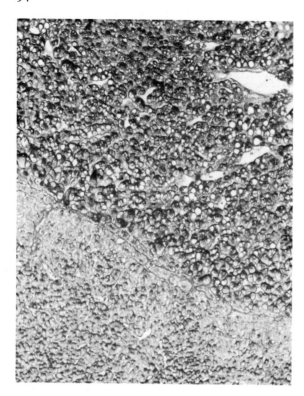

Fig. 29. Cells of HCA contain a far greater quantity of glycogen (*dark part* of photomicrograph) than cells of adjacent parenchyma. AFIP Neg. No. 73-9510, PAS

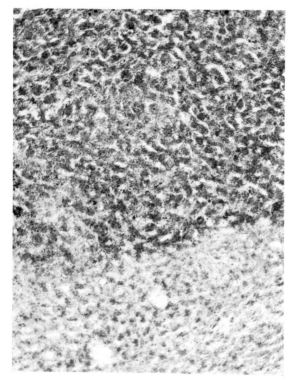

Fig. 30. A moderate quantity of lipid in the form of small droplets is present in the cells of HCA. The adjacent parenchyma (lightly stained *lower third* of photographic field) contains no fat. AFIP Neg. No. 76-10043, Oil-red-0 stain of frozen section, × 60

usually in excess of the quantities found in the non-neoplastic parenchyma of the same liver. In addition to glycogen and fat the cells of HCA may contain bile. Lipofuscin pigment is generally absent (Fig. 31), but occasional tumors may contain some pigment. In many of the tumors elongated, needle-shaped eosinophilic inclusions, presumed to be enlarged mitochondria, can be identified in an otherwise empty cytoplasm. Globular cytoplasmic inclusions that are usually PAS-positive are a very infrequent finding. Mallory's bodies are not seen in the cells of HCA.

The nuclei of cells of HCA usually show little or, less often, moderate variation in size and occupy a relatively small part of the total cell volume (Figs. 26—28). They are normochromatic, have fine or medium-sized chromatin granules and inconspicuous amphophilic nucleoli. Mitotic figures are absent. Most of the cells contain one nucleus, but occasionally cells may contain two or three nuclei; multinucleated cells are exceptionally rare and, when present, have nuclei that do not differ from the single ones described above. Nuclear vacuoles, a frequent finding in hepatocellular carcinoma, are not present in HCA.

Varying-sized areas of recent and old hemorrhage and, less often, infarction are present in the majority of the tumors (Figs. 32—34). The hemorrhages often plough through large areas of the neoplastic parenchyma, with or without rupture; in some cases so much of the tumor is replaced by hemorrhage that the surgeon operating on the patient has difficulty in grossly identifying an underlying tumor. Old hemorrhages show lysis of extravasated erythrocytes and/or fibrin deposition. Much older hemorrhages are represented by poorly vascularized scars that may contain scattered hemosiderin granules (Fig. 33). Recent infarcts consist of sharply defined areas of coagulated neoplastic parenchyma (Fig. 34); these too heal by

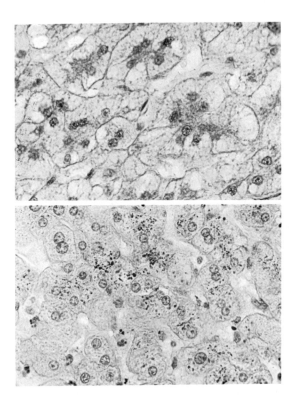

Fig. 31. Cells of HCA (*top*) do not contain lipofuscin, whereas the cells of the adjacent parenchyma (*bottom*) do. AFIP Neg. No. 71-11497, Fontana, × 395

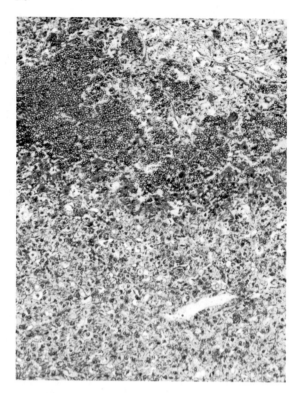

Fig. 32. Recent hemorrhage in HCA. AFIP Neg. No. 71-8102, H & E, × 130

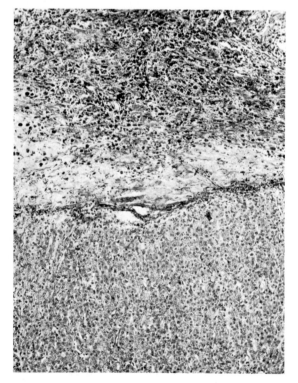

Fig. 33. Area of old hemorrhage (*top half* of field) shows fibrosis and much hemosiderin pigment. AFIP Neg. No. 74-5449, H & E, × 70

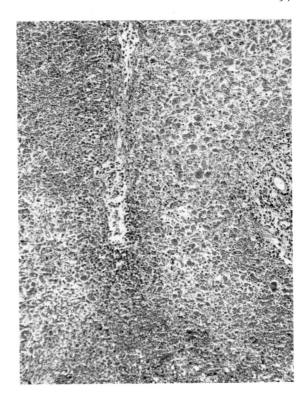

Fig. 34. Infarcted area in HCA.
AFIP Neg. No. 74-5462, H & E,
× 100

fibrosis and often contain hemosiderin and bright yellow hemofuscin pigment. Thrombosis of vessels leading to the infarction may not be evident unless looked for in multiple sections (Fig. 35). It is possible that some of the hemorrhages and/or infarcts are secondary to the vascular changes mentioned above which can compromise the caliber of the lumen without actual thrombosis. EDMONDSON et al. [43] have suggested constriction of arteries supplying HCA as a possible mechanism of necrosis and hemorrhage.

Focal necrosis is a relatively infrequent finding in HCA (Fig. 36). It is probable that much of the "necrosis" grossly described in the AFIP cases (37%) represents infarction or areas of organizing hemorrhage. The foci of necrosis are usually microscopic and are infiltrated by lymphocytes and/or neutrophils. In a few instances noncaseating granulomas have been noted in the HCA but not in the adjacent non-neoplastic parenchyma (Fig. 37).

As noted earlier the majority of patients with HCA have one neoplasm. When multiple tumors are present they generally show similar histologic features. In some patients the liver adjacent to a single large tumor may show occasional microscopic "hyperplastic" foci, the cells of which resemble those of the main tumor. These foci are usually less than the size of an hepatic lobule. Such hyperplastic foci have been commented on by others [20, 28].

The light microscopic features of HCA are compared and contrasted with those of FNH and HCC in Table 4.

The hepatic parenchyma adjacent to HCA may show no changes or a variety of changes. "Acute" changes such as hemorrhages and foci of infarction or necrosis may be seen in livers that contain ruptured tumors. Some of the patients who develop shock may have centrilobular coagulative necrosis of anoxic etiology. "Chronic" alterations include compression atrophy

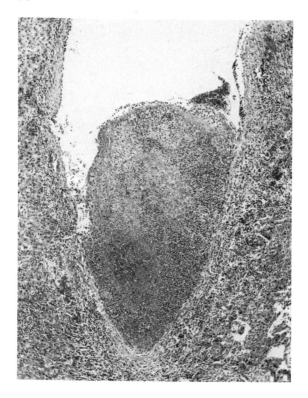

Fig. 35. Thrombosed vein in same HCA illustrated in Figure 34. AFIP Neg. No. 74-5446, H & E, × 50

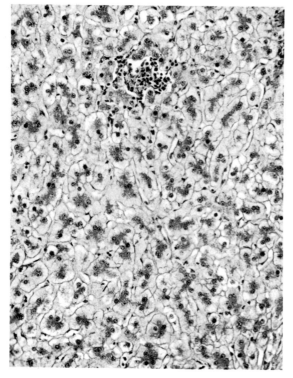

Fig. 36. Small focus of necrosis (*top*) in HCA. AFIP Neg. No. 71-11456, H & E,   195

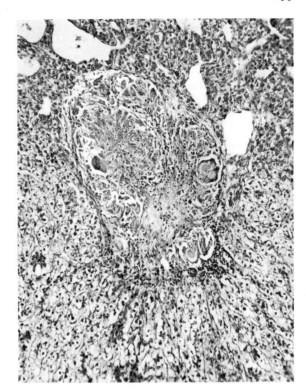

Fig. 37. Noncaseating granuloma within HCA. AFIP Neg. No. 66-1022, H & E, × 100

that is usually directly proportional to the size of the tumor. There may be slight to moderate periportal fibrosis, patchy cholangiolar proliferation, and portal inflammation; these changes progressively diminish as the distance from the tumor increases. Sinusoidal dilatation, sometimes midzonal or periportal, is seen in some of the cases (Fig. 38). The sinusoidal lesions are similar to those reported by WINCKLER and POULSEN [153] in women on OC and also to those produced experimentally in female rats given norethynodrel [13].

The author has not encountered any true case of peliosis hepatis in the non-neoplastic parenchyma of HCA. It is unfortunate that the term "peliosis hepatis" has been used to describe vascular ectasia in HCA and has been considered a feature supporting an etiologic relationship to OC [31]. In the author's experience such a change occurs in most of the tumors regardless of whether or not the patient had taken OC.

No veno-occlusive disease or hepatic vein thrombosis has been noted in the AFIP material, although one such case has been reported [3]. It is also worth noting that no instance of intrahepatic cholestasis has been observed in the AFIP material, nor is the present author aware of any reported cases. With reference to the coexistence of other hepatic neoplasms, one of the AFIP patients also had a FNH, and there are two other examples of this association in the literature [7, 54]. It is of interest that cavernous hemangioma of the liver, a tumor found in association with some cases of FNH, is not known to occur with HCA.

A number of studies of the ultrastructure of HCA have been reported [9, 65, 76, 117]. All studies have emphasized the resemblance of the tumor cells to normal hepatocytes, but the overall structure is greatly "simplified", compared to normal liver cells [117]. One frequent abnormality is the variation in size and shape of mitochondria, with giant mitochondria and

Table 4. Comparison of microscopic features of FNH, HCA, and HCC

Morphologic criterion	FNH	HCA	HCC
Vascular lesions:			
Fibromuscular thickening	Present	Absent	Absent
Subintimal fibrosis	Present	Present	Absent
Intimal hyperplasia	Absent	Present	Absent
Thromboses	Absent	Present or absent	Present or absent
Central stellate scars	Present	Absent	Absent
Septa with bile ducts	Present	Absent	Absent
Inflammation of septa	Present	Absent	Absent
Trabeculae	2-cells thick	2-cells thick	Many cells thick
Reticulin fibers	Well developed	Poorly developed	Poorly developed
Sinusoids	Normal width	Slitlike	Wide and irregular
Canaliculi	Present, normal	Present, may be dilated	Present, may be dilated and bizarre
Canalicular bile plugs	Absent	Present or absent	Present or absent
Hemorrhages	Absent	Present	Present
Infarcts	Absent	Present	Present
Focal necrosis	Present, rare – adjacent to septa ('piecemeal')	Present, rare – small foci	Present, frequent – small or large foci
Extramedullary hematopoiesis	Absent	Present, rare	Absent

	Normal	Larger than normal	Larger or smaller than normal
Cell size	Normal	Larger than normal	Larger or smaller than normal
Anisocytosis	Minimal	Minimal	Marked
Giant cells	Absent	Absent	Present
Cell membrane	Distinct	Distinct	Distinct or ill defined
Cytoplasmic bile	Absent	Present or absent	Present or absent
Cytoplasmic glycogen	Greater than non-neoplastic liver	Greater than non-neoplastic liver	Less or greater than non-neoplastic liver
Cytoplasmic fat	Present or absent	Present or absent	Present or absent
Cytoplasmic acidophilic globules	Absent	Present, rare	Present, frequent
Cytoplasmic Mallory bodies	Absent	Absent	Present, rare
'Ground-glass' tumor cells	Absent	Absent	Present, rare
Cytoplasmic lipofuscin	Absent	Present, rare	Absent
Nuclear size	Normal	Normal or small	Usually large
Anisonucleosis	Minimal	Minimal	Usually marked
Multiple nuclei	Absent	Absent	Present
Chromatin granules	Fine	Fine	Coarse
Nucleoli	Small, amphophilic	Small, amphophilic	Large, acidophilic
Mitoses	Absent	Absent	Present, frequent

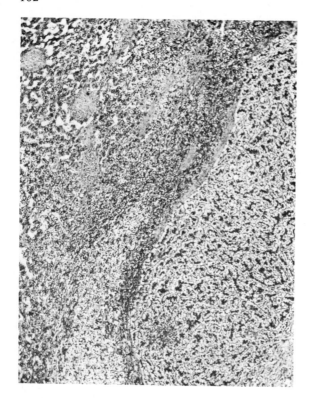

Fig. 38. Parenchyma (*upper and left*) adjacent to HCA shows moderate sinusoidal dilatation in zones 1 and 2 of the Rappaport acinus. AFIP Neg. No. 11-11459, Masson's trichrome, × 50

paracrystalline inclusions (Fig. 39). PHILLIPS et al. [117] could not identify lipofuscin pigment in the cases they studied. BALÁZS [9] specifically commented on the absence of sinusoids and their replacement by capillaries with swollen endothelial cells, pericytes, and a basement membrane. PHILLIPS et al. [117] remarked on the great reduction in the number of bile canaliculi compared to the normal liver. Canaliculi usually occurred at the junction of three hepatocytes (Fig. 40), but occasionally dilated canaliculi were bordered by seven or more hepatocytes. Both KAY and SCHATZKI [76] and BALÁZS [9] identified bile ducts in their cases, despite their apparent absence with light microscopy.

The majority of the patients studied at AFIP underwent surgery following discovery of the HCA. The mortality rate for the entire series was 9%, the major causes of death being hemorrhage and postoperative complications [125]. Of the 32 women who continued to use OC after the first operation, 4 (12.5%) required a second operation because they developed another or recurrent HCA. Other recurrences of HCA have been reported [137]. One of the AFIP patients whose HCA was biopsied but not removed and another whose tumor was only partially resected experienced regression of their tumor after discontinuation of OC. Several cases of regression of HCA following discontinuation of OC [5, 27, 32] have been reported, but it should be emphasized that cessation of OC therapy does not remove the risk of future hemorrhage from HCA [49]. No definite cases of HCC have developed in any of the patients in the AFIP series whose tumors were associated with OC. As noted earlier there is one hepatocellular carcinoma that is thought to have arisen in an HCA [35]. Another case of an HCA with possible transition to HCC has been reported [54]. Other cases of hepatocellular

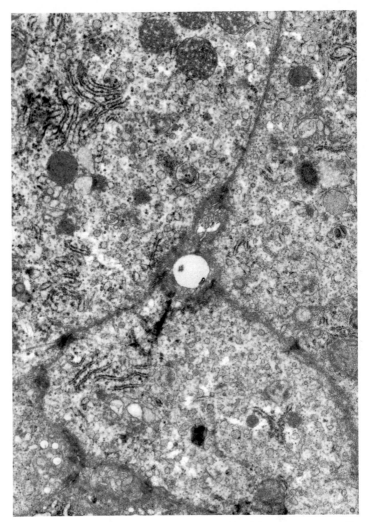

Fig. 39. Electron micrograph of HCA showing central canaliculus bordered by three tumor cells. Note sparsity of profiles of rough endoplasmic reticulum and mitochondria. AFIP Neg. No. 77-8958

carcinoma (and other malignancies) attributed to OC are briefly discussed in another section.

Since the report of BAUM et al. [12] attention has focused on the relationship between HCA and prior use of OC. Before discussion of this association note should be made of the fact that some cases of HCA have been reported in a number of metabolic disorders, such as type I glycogenosis [66] and galactosemia [41]. In addition to these a number of cases have occurred in children [25, 26, 28, 34, 69, 110, 118, 140, 152]. As will be noted later some of the tumors associated with anabolic steroids have been classified as HCA or "benign hepatoma" [22, 86, 139]. Also, a considerable number of published cases (138 cases according to the review of KLATSKIN [79]) of HCA had had no history of exposure to OC.

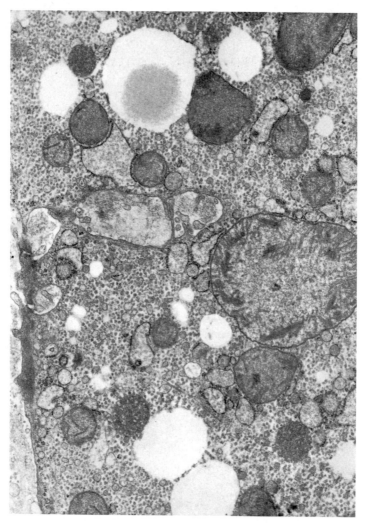

Fig. 40. Electron micrograph of cytoplasm of a tumor cell of an HCA shows marked variation in size of mitochondria; one megamitochondrion (*center, right*) shows an increased number of atypically oriented cristae. The smooth endoplasmic reticulum is increased, whereas only a few dilated cisterns of rough endoplasmic reticulum are seen. The cytoplasm is full of glycogen and contains a number of empty spaces representing lipid. A large vacuole (*top*) contains a slightly dense material with a fuzzy outline resembling α_1-antitrypsin. A canaliculus (*center, left*) contains some fibrillar material probably representing bile. AFIP Neg. No. 77-8959

The absolute incidence of HCA in patients on OC has not been established. In the state of Iowa, U.S.A., the incidence has been estimated to be 0.29 per 100,000 women per year [17]. Another estimate by BAUM [11] places the incidence between 1 : 500,000 to 1 : 1,000,000 women taking OC. The majority of cases of HCA have been reported from the United States. Several long-term follow-up studies of women on OC from Great Britain (Royal College of General Practitioners, Oxford Family Planning Association, and other data bases) have shown only a single benign tumor ("hamartoma") of the liver [75, 112, 149]. Two case-control studies have been conducted in the United States. EDMONDSON et al. [43] found a significant difference between cases and matched controls in mean months of OC use: 73.4 as compared to 36.2 (P < 0.001). The relative risk increased dramatically with duration of use, particularly after 60 months. In the study conducted by the AFIP and Center for Disease Control (C.D.C.), Atlanta, Georgia, the risk of developing HCA is estimated to be 9, 120, and 500 times higher, respectively for women with less than 4, 4–7, and 8 or more years of OC use [125]. EDMONDSON et al. [43] reported that women with HCA took OC containing mestranol much more commonly than controls (P < 0.0001). Their conclusion of a greater risk of HCA developing with the use of OC composed mainly of mestranol (as opposed to those containing ethinylestradiol) has been questioned by others [79]. In the AFIP-C.D.C. study no meaningful difference was determined between cases and controls in regards to the type of synthetic estrogen contained in the OC used [125]. However, a definite relationship was revealed between hormonal potency of the OC composition and the risk of development of HCA, the higher potency formulations being associated with a greater risk than those of lower potency, for comparable durations of use. In addition to duration of use and hormonal potency of the contraceptive steroid, a woman's age affects her chances of developing HCA. Thus, women less than 27 years of age had no more than 20-fold increases in the risk of developing HCA irrespective of the length of use of OC.

Conflicting results have been reported on the induction of tumors by OC in animal species; these studies have recently been summarized [123]. An increased incidence of "regenerative nodules" and HCA have been reported in albino rats receiving norethindrone acetate plus ethinylestradiol over a 104-week period [129]. Others have not shown such an increase [96]. No liver tumors have been observed, however, in dogs and monkeys on long-term OC [15, 83, 150].

Nodular Regenerative Hyperplasia

This condition was first described by Steiner [135] in 1959 who stated that "hepatocytic hyperplasia or regeneration may take place in the absence of fibrous tissue proliferation, that it may be nodular, and that the resulting lesion, here called nodular regenerative hyperplasia, may simulate cirrhosis without, however, meeting the precise criteria and definition of "cirrhosis". STEINER's observations were based on a study of 12 autopsy cases, but the details of the cases were not mentioned. However, he also stated that the condition was "associated with a variety of major diseases, the commonest of which have been the passive congestion of severe heart failure and tuberculosis".

Although rare, NRH has been reported subsequently by a number of authors [19, 29, 30, 36, 58, 82, 88, 89, 122, 130]. It is also known as partial nodular transformation of the liver, nodular transformation of the liver, nodular, noncirrhotic liver, and regenerative nodular hyperplasia of the liver. The condition has been reported in patients with Felty's syndrome, rheumatoid arthritis, CRST syndrome (calcinosis cutis, Raynaud's phenomenon, sclerodactylia and telangiectasia), or may be idiopathic. Also, as noted in another section, some cases of HCA with multiple tumors may show foci that resemble those of NRH, a finding also observed by others [21, 28]. The occurrence of NRH in three patients treated with anabolic steroids [127, 139], one of whom also had an HCA [139], is noted in the next section.

The gross appearance of NRH is highly characteristic. The hyperplastic foci arise in a noncirrhotic parenchyma, are distributed throughout the liver, and vary from less than 1 mm to 1 cm or more in diameter; only the larger lesions are "nodular". In some cases the nodules may be clustered in the area around the porta hepatis [128]. The lesions are sharply demarcated but nonencapsulated, and are off-white, light tan, yellowish-brown, or even yellow in color. They are often seen more clearly after formalin fixation than in the fresh state.

Microscopically, the smaller lesions of NRH merge almost imperceptibly with the surrounding parenchyma, but the larger lesions may cause compression (Fig. 41). The lesions may be smaller than an hepatic lobule or may be equivalent in size to multiple lobules. They usually do not have a "substructure" (i.e., they do not contain central veins or portal areas). Occasional nodules may, however, incorporate preexisting portal areas or central veins; this may occur by the confluence of several adjacent hyperplastic foci. Reticulum stains are especially useful in "mapping out" the lesions because of the thicker plates, the different orientation of the plates from those of the rest of the lobule, and the compression, however slight, of the neighboring parenchyma (Fig. 42). Some connective tissue, usually in the form of fine septa surrounding part of the circumference of the larger nodules, may be demonstrable by special stains for collagen. Sinusoids in the adjacent parenchyma, and sometimes within the lesions, may be dilated.

The hepatocytes comprising the nodules are arranged in plates two-cells thick with canaliculi between them. The canaliculi may be dilated with formation of pseudoglands, but they only rarely contain bile. Sinusoids between the plates are slitlike and their lining cells are flat. The

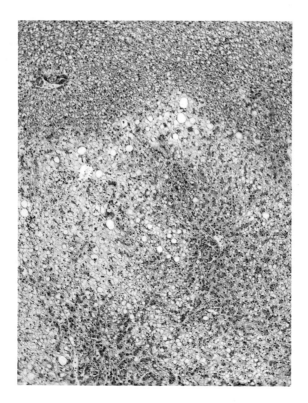

Fig. 41. Lesion of NRH is sharply demarcated from the adjacent parenchyma (*top*) but is nonencapsulated. AFIP Neg. No. 76-11882, H & E, × 60

cells are larger than normal hepatocytes and usually have a lightly eosinophilic of empty ("clear") cytoplasm (Figs. 43 and 44). Some cells contain lipid vacuoles in the cytoplasm and in some cases almost all the component cells are vacuolated (Figs. 41, 43, and 44). The pallor of the cytoplasm can be shown to be the result of accumulation of glycogen, often in excess of that in the adjacent parenchyma (Fig. 45), whereas the vacuoles are sudanophilic in frozen sections (Fig. 46). The lesions may be composed of either clear or vacuolated cells or an admixture of both. If hemosiderin is present in the adjacent parenchyma none can be demonstrated in the lesions. Also, lipofuscin pigment that is normally present in the adjacent parenchyma, cannot be identified in the cells of NRH. Bile retention, either cytoplasmic or canalicular, is rarely present. The nuclei are usually larger than those of the normal hepato- prominent amphophilic or eosinophilic nucleoli. STEINER [135] noted that mitotic figures may occasionally be present. Many of the cells contain two or three nuclei.

Although the aforementioned features bear some resemblance to those of HCA, the cytologic features, particularly the nuclear characteristics, are more in keeping with those of the cells of regenerative nodules in precirrhotic, e.g., chronic active hepatitis with nodular regeneration or in cirrhotic livers. The association with the previously mentioned diseases, particularly the "collagen diseases" of NRH together with its almost invariable association with portal hypertension are further clinical differences that distinguish that entity from HCA. While NRH may be premalignant, the development of HCC has yet to be convincingly demon- strated in a single case.

The lesions in NRH in humans do resemble those that occur spontaneously in animals or are experimentally induced by a wide variety of carcinogens (e.g., ethionine, aflatoxin B, 2-

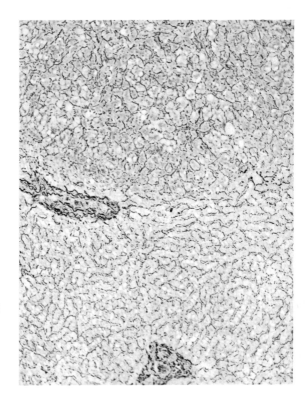

Fig. 42. Reticulum network of NRH (*upper half* of field) shows thicker plates and a different orientation of the fibers from the parenchyma below. AFIP Neg. No. 76-11893, Manuel's reticulum, × 80

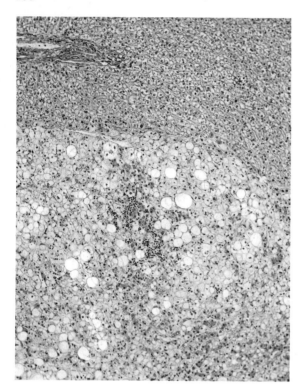

Fig. 43. Cells of NRH are larger and paler than those of nearby hepatic parenchyma (*top*). Some contain medium and large lipid vacuoles. A focus of necrosis is present in the NRH. AFIP Neg. No. 76-1180, H & E, × 80

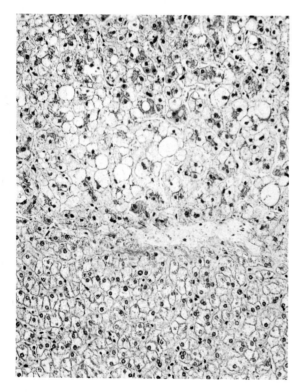

Fig. 44. Cells of NRH are large, pale, and vacuolated. The nuclei are about the same size as those of the normal parenchyma *below*. AFIP Neg. No. 76-11898, H & E, × 165

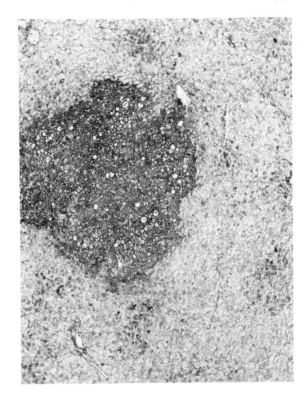

Fig. 45. Cells of NRH are darkly stained because of their large content of glycogen. AFIP Neg. No. 76-11892, PAS, × 50

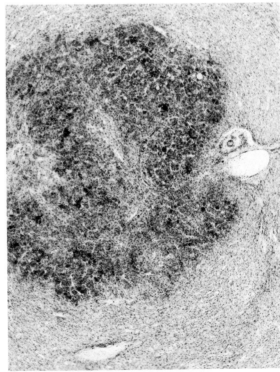

Fig. 46. Sharply defined NRH shows dark cells filled with fine lipid droplets. AFIP Neg. No. 76-11889, Frozen section stained with oil-red-0, × 60

acetylaminofluorene). SCHARDEIN et al. [129] have produced such lesions in rats given OC. The terms "hyperplastic foci", "hyperplastic liver nodules", and "neoplastic foci" have been used for the lesions in animals [47, 132]. Despite the microscopic similarities between the human and animal lesions, acidophilic or "ground-glass" cells or atypical basophilic cells (the latter considered to be malignant) have not been observed by the present author in human cases, nor have they heretofore been described in published reports. Altered patterns of isoenzymes (such as low glucose-6-phosphatase or adenosinetriphosphatase activities) have yet to be demonstrated in human cases. Finally, no studies for presence or absence of α-fetoprotein, α_1-antitrypsin, or preneoplastic antigen [47] have been performed in human cases. Whether or not all human cases of HCA and HCC associated with OC or AS go through a stage of NRH must still be determined, although it remains a distinct possibility, as suggested by LINGEMAN [87].

Hepatocellular Carcinoma and Other Malignancies

The reported cases of malignant hepatic tumors in patients who had been taking OC are listed in Table 5. One case that was initially reported as an HCC [63] was, on subsequent review, apparently considered to be an HCA [49]. In addition to the four cases of HCC in women on OC published by MAYS et al. [94] another five cases are mentioned by these authors in subsequent publications [27, 28]. These other cases are not included in Table 5 because data on the individual cases were not mentioned. The total number of reported cases of malignant hepatic tumors in patients taking contraceptive steroids is therefore 16, 14 of which were classified as HCC, one as a combined bile duct and hepatocellular carcinoma [115], and one as a mixed hepatoblastoma [100]. The duration of use of OC prior to diagnosis was less than 1 year in three patients and up to 2 years in seven patients. The average "latent period" was 45.3 months (figure based on cases listed in Table 5 only).

The clinical presentations of the patients with malignant tumors do not differ significantly from those of patients who had not received OC. A serum α-fetoprotein determination was performed in 4 of the 11 cases and was positive in only 1 case [141]. Of the 11 patients 5 were dead and 6 alive at the time of publication. Only one of the deceased patients was autopsied, but no evidence of extrahepatic metastases was found [120].

A relationship between HCC as well as other malignant tumors of the liver and prior use of OC has not been determined. The duration of use of OC in some of the published cases seems unduly short, as previously noted by HENDERSON et al. [60], when compared to the latent period of other known hepatocarcinogens such as thorotrast or vinyl chloride ($\sim$ 14–20 years). Mortality from primary cancer of the liver has changed little among women in the United States from 1958 to 1975 [124], in contrast to the remarkable increase in the number of hepatocellular adenomas after 1960. Despite the aforementioned "negative" evidence a relationship between malignant tumors of the liver and OC cannot be entirely dismissed because of their occurrence in patients on anabolic steroids and the possible role of endogenous estrogens in the etiology of HCC [26, 33]. Also, as noted in the section on HCA, a few cases of apparently malignant transformation of benign tumors in patients on OC have been reported. The small number of cases of HCC in women taking OC has so far hampered epidemiologic case-control studies similar to those conducted in patients with HCA. The reporting of more cases in the coming years should provide more insight into any etiologic role of OC in HCC.

Table 5. Malignant tumors associated with oral contraceptives

Author(s) (years)	Reference	Age	Type of oral contraceptive[a]	Duration (mo.)	Clinical	Management and course	Pathologic diagnosis
Thalassinos et al. (1974)	141	30	Drugs with estrogen activity Clomiphene	42 3	Fever. Chills, subcostal pain. Hepatosplenomegaly. Hepatic scan +	Laparotomy and biopsy. Postoperative chemotherapy. Alive	HCC
Meyer et al. (1974)	100	19	Norethindrone + mestranol	15	Fever. Abdominal pain. Hepatosplenomegaly. α-fetoprotein − Arteriogram: Avascular mass. Hepatic scan +	Lobectomy, right. Alive	Hepatoblastoma, mixed type
Davis et al. (1975)	35	21	4 mg megestrol acetate 50 μg ethinyl − estradiol	24	Anemia. Hepatomegaly. α-fetoprotein − HBsAG − Hepatic scan +	Lobectomy, left. Alive	HCC arising in FNH
Mays et al. (1976)	94	47	N.R.	12	Right shoulder pain. Abdominal pain. Shock. Hemoperitoneum	Lobectomy, right. Died at operation	HCC
Mays et al. (1976)	94	25	N.R.	6	Epigastric mass, rapidly enlarging	Laparatomy and biopsy. Died	HCC
Mays et al. (1976)	94	25	Norgestrel + mestranol	12	Epigastric mass. Mild discomfort in upper abdomen	Laparatomy and biopsy. Died	HCC
Mays et al. (1976)	94	25	Norgestrel + mestranol	60	Multiple admissions for sporadic left-pleuritic pain (6 yrs.). Severe constant right-pleuritic pain (1 mo.)	Lobectomy, right. Alive, 2 mo.	HCC

Table 5. (continued)

Author(s) (years)	Reference	Age	Type of oral contraceptive[a]	Duration (mo.)	Clinical	Management and course	Pathologic diagnosis
O'Sullivan and Rossiwck (1976)	115	44	N.R.	24	Epigastric pain. Anorexia. Malaise, weight loss. Hepatomegaly. Ultrasound: massive hepatomegaly with replacement by malignant masses.	Laparotomy and biopsy. Postoperative chemotherapy. Alive.	HCC and bile duct carcinoma
Glassberg and Rosenbaum (1976)	53	31	1 mg norethisterone + 0.8 mg mestranol. 2 mg northisterone + 0.1 mg mestranol	60 72	Abdominal pain. Epigastric mass. Hepatic scan +	Laparotomy and biopsy. Postoperative chemotherapy. Alive.	HCC
Tigano et al. (1976)	144	32	2,5 mg lynestrenol + 75 µg mestranol	24	Dull ache, right hypochondrium. Fever. Jaundice. Hepatosplenomegaly. Alpha fetoprotein + Hepatic scan +	Laparotomy and biopsy. Died	HCC
Pryor et al. (1977)	120	32	5 mg norethynodrel + 0.075 mg mestranol for 8 years. 1 mg norethindrone + 0.08 mg mestranol for 4 years	144	Sporadic epigastric and right upper quadrant pain (9 mo.). Alpha fetoprotein − Hepatic scan +	Laparotomy and biopsy. Postoperative chemotherapy. Died	HCC No metastases at autopsy

[a] — N.R. = not reported; + = positive test or procedure; − = negative test or procedure.

Tumors and Tumorlike Lesions of the Liver Associated with Anabolic-Androgenic Steroids

Twenty-two cases of tumors and tumorlike lesions of the liver have been reported in patients on long-term therapy with C-17 alkylated androgenic-anabolic steroids. These together with two additional cases in the AFIP files are summarized in Table 6. Thirteen of the patients were in the pediatric age range at the time of onset of the disease for which anabolic steroids were prescribed. Nineteen were males and five were females. The dosage and duration of therapy (2—360 months, average 67.65 months) with the various anabolic steroids given prior to the discovery of the hepatic tumors varied widely. An exceptionally long "latent period" of 24 years was recorded in one patient with Fanconi's anemia [57] following a short course of therapy. Doubts regarding a relationship between the anabolic steroids and the subsequent development of a hepatocellular carcinoma have been expressed by these authors [57] and others [72]. Two other cases [103, 139] were exposed to anabolic steroids for a very short period of time — 2 and 3 months, respectively; one [136] had hyperplastic hepatic nodules and the other [103], HCC. Although these two cases are included in the table such a short "latent period" again casts doubt on an etiologic relationship between the hepatic tumors and the anabolic steroids.

The majority of the patients (19 of the 24) had been treated for various types of anemia, nine with Fanconi's anemia. At least half the patients had also received multiple blood transfusions.

Physical findings pertaining to involvement of the liver included hepatomegaly (13 patients), an upper abdominal mass (2 patients), and jaundice (6 patients). Two patients presented with an acute abdomen due to rupture of the tumor. Stigmata of chronic hepatic disease (spider nevi, palmar erythema, etc.) were evident in four patients.

Sixteen of the patients had abnormal results from tests of hepatic function. Alpha-fetoprotein was detected in the serum from only 2 of the 17 patients tested; one of these patients was also seropositive for HBsAg.

Hepatic scans were performed in 15 patients. Four were normal, ten showed an area or areas of decreased radioactive uptake (with or without hepatomegaly), while one showed a diffuse infiltrative process. Arteriograms were performed in three patients, one, postmortem; one showed a "tumor mass" [155], the second showed displacement of vessels by a mass [108], and two showed an abnormal circulation in the right lobe (Case 1 of SWEENEY and EVANS [139]; PORT et al. [119]).

Only 6 of the 24 patients were alive when the case reports were published. Two of the patients of FARRELL et al. [48] were alive 4 and 7 years after detection of their hepatic neoplasia, but one showed evidence of osseous metastases. Both of these patients, as well as another patient (Case 1 of JOHNSON et al. [73]), had shown evidence of tumor regression following cessation of anabolic steroid therapy. Of the 18 patients who died 9 did so from internal hemorrhages (gastrointestinal, intracranial, etc.); one patient bled intraperitoneally from rupture of a liver adenoma [86]. Four patients died from liver failure [18, 119, 139]. Other causes of death were sepsis [127] and carcinomatosis [103]. The cause of death in three patients was unknown [61, 73, 78].

All but one [61] of the cases were histologically confirmed. Five of the cases were classified as benign (hyperplastic nodules, HCA), whereas the rest were interpreted as HCC. More carcinomas (11 cases) were multicentric than unicentric (5 cases). One patient had vascular invasion by the tumor [119], whereas two patients had distant metastases [48, 103]. The difficulties in diagnosis of the hepatocellular tumors associated with the anabolic steroids

Table 6. Summary of reported tumors associated with anabolic steroids

Author(s) (year)	Reference	Sex/age[a]	Diagnosis	Drug	Dosage (mg/day)[b]	Duration (months)	Trans-fusions
Bernstein et al. (1971)	(18)	M/20	Fanconi's anemia	Oxymetholone	100	100	−
Port et al. (1971)	(119)	M/21	Fanconi's anemia	Oxymetholone	?	9	−
Johnson et al. (1972)	(72)	F/2½	Aplastic anemia	Oxymetholone	30–100	46	+
Johnson et al. (1972)	(72)	F/17	Aplastic anemia	Oxymetholone	150–250	28	+
Recant and Lacey (1965) Johnson et al. (1972)	(121) (73)	M/14	Fanconi's anemia	Methyltestosterone	20	40	+
Johnson et al. (1972)	(73)	M/21	Fanconi's anemia	Methandrostenolone	10–50	89	−
Zeigenfuss and Carabasi (1973)	(155)	M/68	"Potency problem"	Methyltestosterone	?	360	−
Henderson et al. (1973)	(61)	M/4	Hypoplastic anemia	Methyltestosterone Norethandrolone Oxymetholone Stanozolol	40–80 10 100 15	21 3 35 18	+
Meadows et al. (1974)	(99)	F/2	Aplastic anemia	Oxymetholone Nandrolone decanoate	60 50 (per week)	41 6	+
Farrell et al. (1975)	(48)	M/28	Paroxysmal nocturnal hemoglobinuria	Oxymetholone	100–150	6	+
Farrell et al. (1975)	(48)	M/40	Hypopituitarism Alcoholism	Methyltestosterone	25–50	20	−
Farrell et al. (1975)	(48)	M/38	Cryptorchidism	Methyltestosterone Testosterone propionate	50 50 (per month)	96 96	−
Mulvihill et al. (1975)	(108)	M/8½	Fanconi's anemia	Oxymetholone	20–60	37	−

Author (year)	Reference	Sex/Age	Diagnosis	Steroid	Dose	[a]	[b]
Holder et al. (1975)	(64)	M/4	Acquired hypoplastic anemia	Methandrostenolone / Oxymetholone / Fluoxymesterone / Nandrolone decanoate	? / ? / ? / 50 (per week)	2 / 13 / ?	+
Bruguera (1975)	(22)	M/16	Paroxysmal nocturnal hemoglobinuria	Oxymetholone	?	36	?
Sarna et al. (1975)	(128)	M/10	Fanconi's anemia	Norethandrolone / Oxandrolone / Oxymetholone	56.7 g (total) / 2.1 g (total) / 1.2 g (total)	88	+
Lesna et al. (1976)	(86)	M/2	Aplastic anemia	Testosterone / Oxymetholone	? / 68	? / ?	+
Sweeney and Evans (1976)	(139)	M/5	Fanconi's anemia	Methyltestosterone / Oxymetholone / Nandrolone decanoate	20 / ? / 25 (per week)	36 / ? / 12	+
Sweeney and Evans (1976)	(139)	M/46	Aplastic anemia	Oxymetholone	100–300	3	−
Kew et al. (1976)	(78)	F/12	Fanconi's anemia	Methyltestosterone / Depo-testosterone and ethinylestradiol / Methyltestosterone / Oxymetholone	100 / 100 / 0.02 / 20 / 150	12 / 9 / 24 / 48	+
Mokrohisky et al. (1977)	(103)	F/6½	Fanconi's anemia	Oxymetholone	?	2	−
Sale and Lerner (1977)	(127)	M/37	Aplastic anemia	Testosterone / Oxymetholone / Methyltestosterone / Fluoxymesterone	? / 100–150 / 75 / ?	35 / ? / ? / ?	+
AFIP Case 1 (1977)	—	M/5	Aplastic anemia	Methyltestosterone / Oxymetholone	70 / 70–210	60 / 24	+
AFIP Case 2 (1977)	—	M/2	Sideroblastic anemia	Oxymetholone	?	60	+

[a] — Age at the time of onset of diagnosis, in years.
[b] — Unless otherwise indicated; + = given; − = not given.

Table 6. (continued)

Author(s)	Reference	Abnormal tests of liver function[a]	Tests for alpha-feto-protein[a]	Tests for HBAg[a]	Type of pathologic material	Pathologic diagnosis of tumor(s)	Pathology of non-neoplastic liver	Metastases or vascular invasion
Bernstein et al. (1971)	(18)	+	N.R.	N.R.	Autopsy	HCC, multicentric	Peliosis hepatis	—
Port et al. (1971)	(119)	N.R.	—	—	Autopsy	HCC, multiple	Peliosis hepatis	Vascular invasion
Johnson et al. (1972)	(73)	—	+	N.R.	Biopsy	HCC, multicentric	Normal	—
Johnson et al. (1972)	(73)	+	—	—	Biopsy and autopsy	HCC, multicentric	Cholestasis Hemosiderosis	—
Recant and Lacey (1965) Johnson et al. (1972)	(121)	+	N.R.	N.R.	Autopsy	HCC, multicentric	Postnecrotic cirrhosis	—
Johnson et al. (1972)	(73)	+	—	N.R.	Biopsy	HCC	N.R. autopsy	No
Zeigenfuss and Carabasi (1973)	(155)	+	—	—	Resected specimen	HCC, single mass	N.R.	—
Henderson et al. (1973)	(61)	+	+	+	None	HCC (presumptive diagnosis)	N.R.	—
Meadows et al. (1974)	(99)	—	N.R.	—	Autopsy	HCC, single mass	Peliosis hepatis	—
Farrell et al. (1975)	(48)	+	—	—	Biopsy	HCC, multicentric	N.R.	—
Farrell et al. (1975)	(48)	+	—	—	Resected specimen	HCC, multicentric	Normal	—

								Ribb and other
Farrell et al. (1975)	(48)	−	−	N.R.	Biopsy	HCC, single mass	Normal metastases	−
Mulvihill et al. (1975)	(108)	+	−	−	Autopsy	HCA, single mass	Normal	−
Holder et al. (1975)	(64)	+	−	−	Autopsy	HCC, single mass	Hemosiderosis	−
Bruguera (1975)	(22)	N.R.	N.R.	N.R.	Resected specimen	HCA, ruptured	N.R.	−
Sarna et al. (1975)	(128)	+	−	−	Autopsy Cholestasis	HCC, multiple	Congestion	−
Lesna et al. (1976)	(86)	N.R.	N.R.	N.R.	Autopsy	HCA, multiple	Hemosiderosis	−
Sweeney and Evans (1976)	(139)	+	−	N.R.	Autopsy	HCA	Generalized hyperplasia with nodule formation. Hemosiderosis	−
Sweeney and Evans (1976)	(139)	+	N.R.	N.R.	Autopsy	Hyperplastic nodules	Cholestasis	−
Kew et al. (1976)	(78)	+	−	N.R.	Biopsy	HCC, multiple	Hemosiderosis	−
Mokrohisky et al. (1977)	(103)	N.R.	−	N.R.	Biopsy	HCC	Normal	Lungs
Sale and Lerner (1977)	(127)	+	−	−	Autopsy	Multiple well-differentiated hepatomas	Hemosiderosis	−
AFIP Case I (1977)	−	+	N.R.	N.R.	Autopsy	HCC, multicentric	Hemosiderosis	−
AFIP Case 2 (1977)	−	+	−	−	Resected specimen	HCC, single mass	Hemosiderosis	−

a − N.R. = not reported; + = present, positive or abnormal; − = absent or negative.

have been commented on by ANTHONY [6] and SWEENEY and EVANS [138]. These difficulties will not be resolved until more cases that are better documented, particularly histologically, are published.

Microscopic study of AFIP Case 1 showed varying-sized tumor nodules scattered through-out the liver, sometimes surrounded by a pseudocapsule and irregularly dissected by fibrous septa (Fig. 47). The reticulum framework of the tumor was poorly developed (Fig. 48), but all the nodules showed striking pseudogland formation (Figs. 49 and 50). This was caused by marked dilatation of canaliculi that were centrally placed in the trabeculae; most of the canalicular lumens contained bile plugs (Figs. 49 and 50). The tumor cells were moderately well differentiated (Fig. 51). Several of the published cases also showed a prominent pseudo-gland pattern [48, 99], as did one of the benign tumors [139]. AFIP Case 2 also showed a tumor mass subdivided into smaller nodules by fibrous septa; these did not contain bile ducts but were infiltrated by inflammatory cells. Trabeculae were small and appeared to be separated by capillaries instead of sinusoids. Pseudogland formation was prominent in many areas and bile was noted in canaliculi and the cytoplasm of tumor cells. Tumor cells were moderately well differentiated and mitoses were rare. Vascular invasion was not noted in this or the other AFIP case.

Changes in the non-neoplastic livers are worth noting for comparison with hepatocellular tumors associated with other "etiologic" factors. In five of the cases of HCC the adjacent liver is not mentioned, whereas in five it was histologically normal. There was only one cirrhotic liver ("postnecrotic" cirrhosis) associated with a hepatocellular carcinoma [73, 121]. Other changes in the non-neoplastic parenchyma included marked hemosiderosis (eight cases)

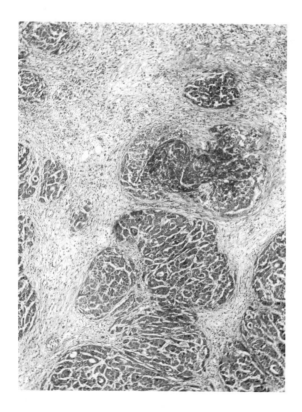

Fig. 47. Tumor nodules of variable size are separated by fibrous tissue. AFIP Neg. No. 76-11944, H & E, × 50

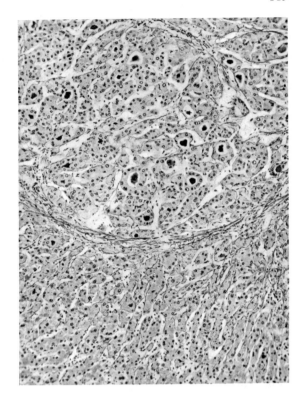

Fig. 48. Tumor nodule (*top*) shows a small trabecular pattern, pseudoglands but only a few supporting reticulum fibers. AFIP Neg. No. 76-11950, Manuel's reticulum, × 80

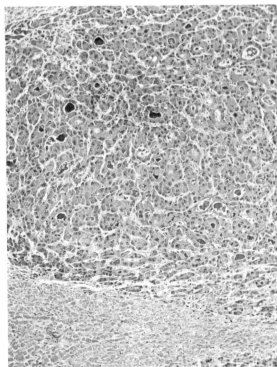

Fig. 49. Small trabeculae of tumor show frequent pseudogland formation. Tumor nodule is well defined but is not separated from the parenchyma *below* by a capsule. AFIP Neg. No. 76-11951, H & E, × 80

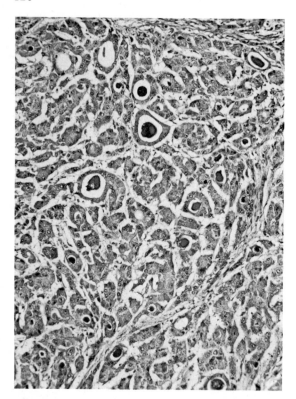

Fig. 50. Pseudogland formation is due to marked dilatation of the canaliculus in the trabeculae. Most of the canaliculi contain bile plugs. AFIP Neg. No. 76-11956, H & E, × 110

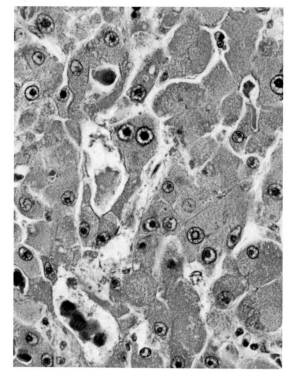

Fig. 51. Cells of HCA show large hyperchromatic nuclei with very prominent nucleoli. Note bile in dilated canaliculi. AFIP Neg. No. 76-11960, H & E, × 440

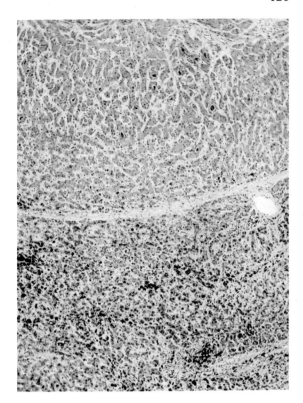

Fig. 52. Hepatic parenchyma (*bottom half* of field) shows marked hemosiderosis. Note absence of hemosiderin in tumor nodule in *top half* of field. AFIP Neg. No. 76-11947, Mallory's stain for iron, × 50

(Fig. 52), peliosis hepatis (three cases), and cholestasis (three cases). (Peliosis hepatis is, of course, a recognized complication of anabolic steroid therapy; NADELL and KOSEK [109] recently reported 12 cases, together with a review of the literature.) No mention of the non-neoplastic parenchyma is made in the case published by BRUGUERA [22]. All patients with hemosiderosis had received multiple blood transfusions.

A definite etiologic relationship between the androgenic-anabolic steroids and hepatocellular tumors and tumorlike lesions remains to be established. Such a relationship is supported by experimental work, recently summarized by JOHNSON [72], and by the clinical resolution of the hepatic tumors in several patients following withdrawal of therapy [48, 72, 73]. Other cofactors may be important since hepatocellular carcinoma has been reported in a patient with Fanconi's anemia [24] and another patient with congenital hypoplastic anemia [136]. Such factors could include an inherent predisposition to the development of neoplasms, e.g., in Fanconi's anemia as pointed out by CATTAN et al. [24] and MOKROHISKY et al. [103], transfusional hemosiderosis [136], viral hepatitis (type B or type "non-A, non-B"), and other drugs (administered simultaneously or before or after the anabolic steroids).

Addendum

After preparation of this review another case of Fanconi's anemia with hepatocellular tumors was published (P. SHAPIRO et al.: Multiple hepatic tumors and peliosis hepatis in Fanconi's anemia treated with androgens. Amer. J. Dis. Child. *131*, 1104—1131, 1977). The patient, a

13-year-old boy, had been treated with androgens and corticosteroids for 5 years. In addition to the hepatocellular tumors, some of which were classified as HCC, the liver showed peliosis hepatis.

References

1. Aldinger, K., Ben-Menachem , Y., Whalen, G.: Focal nodular hyperplasia of the liver associated with high-dosage estrogens. Arch. Intern. Med. *137*, 357–359 (1977)
2. Alpert, E.: Human alpha-1 fetoprotein. In: Hepatocellular Carcinoma. Okuda, K. and Peters, R. L. (Eds.). New York: John Wiley and Sons, 1976a, pp. 353–367
3. Alpert, L. I.: Veno-occlusive disease of the liver associated with oral contraceptives. Hum. Pathol. *7*, 709–718 (1976b)
4. Ameriks, J. A., Thompson, N. W., Frey, C. F., Appelman, H. D., Walter, J. F.: Hepatic cell adenomas, spontaneous liver rupture, and oral contraceptives. Arch. Surg. *110*, 548–556 (1975)
5. Andersen, P. H., Packer, J. T.: Hepatic adenoma. Observations after estrogen withdrawal. Arch. Surg. *111*, 898–900 (1976)
6. Anthony, P. P.: Hepatoma associated with androgenic steroids. Lancet *1*, 685–686 (1975)
7. Antoniades, K., Campbell, W. N., Hecksher, R. H., Kessler, W. B., McCarthy, G. E., Jr.: Liver cell adenoma and oral contraceptives. Double tumor development. JAMA *234*, 628–629 (1975)
8. Baek, S., Sloane, C. E., Futterman, S. C.: Benign liver cell adenoma associated with use of oral contraceptive agents. Ann. Surg. *183*, 239–242 (1976)
9. Balázs, M.: Electron microscopic study of benign hepatoma in a patient on oral contraceptives. Beitr. Pathol. Bd. *159*, 299–306 (1976)
10. Bartók, I., Garas, S., Szabó, L.: Oral contraceptives and benign liver tumour. Lancet *1*, 478–479 (1976)
11. Baum, J. K.: Liver tumors and oral contraceptives. JAMA *232*, 1329 (1975)
12. Baum, J. K., Holtz, F., Bookstein, J. J., Klein, E. W.: Possible association between benign hepatomas and oral contraceptives. Lancet *2*, 926–929 (1973)
13. Beaconsfield, P.: Liver tumours and steroid hormones. Lancet *1*, 516–517 (1974)
14. Begg, C. F., Berry, W. H.: Isolated nodules of regenerative hyperplasia of the liver. Am. J. Clin. Pathol. *27*, 447–463 (1953)
15. Belavady, B., Krishnamurthi, D., Mohiuddin, S. M., Rao, P. U.: Metabolic effects of oral contraceptives in monkeys fed adequate protein and low protein diets. Indian J. Exp. Biol. *11*, 15–22 (1973)
16. Benz, E. J., Baggenstoss, A. H.: Focal cirrhosis of the liver. Its relation to the so-called hamartoma (adenoma, benign hepatoma). Cancer *6*, 743–755 (1953)
17. Berg, J. W., Ketelaar, R. J., Rose, E. F., Vernon, R. G.: Hepatomas and oral contraceptives. Lancet *2*, 349–350 (1974)
18. Bernstein, M. S., Hunter, R. L., Yachnin, S.: Hepatoma and peliosis hepatis developing in a patient with Fanconi's anemia. New Engl. J. Med. *284*, 1135–1136 (1971)
19. Blendis, L. M., Parkinson, M. C., Shilkin, K. B., Williams, R.: Nodular regenerative hyperplasia of the liver in Felty's syndrome. Q. J. Med. *169*, 25–32 (1974)
20. Brander, W., Bewick, M., Ogg, C.: Liver hamartomas in patients on oral contraceptives. Br. Med. J. *2*, 80 (1974)
21. Brander, W. L., Vosnides, G., Ogg, C. S., West, I. E.: Multiple hepatocellular tumours in a patient treated with oral contraceptives. Virchows Arch. *370*, 69–76 (1976)
22. Bruguera, M.: Hepatoma associated with androgenic steroids. Lancet *1*, 1295 (1975)

23. Catalano, P. W., Early, M. E., Topolosky, H. W., Martin, E. W., Jr., Carey, L. C.: Focal nodular hyperplasia of the liver. Report of six patients. Concepts of surgical management. Cancer *39*, 587–591 (1977)

24. Cattan, D., Vesin, P., Wautier, J., Khalifat, R., Meignan, S.: Liver tumours and steroid hormones. Lancet *1*, 878 (1974)

25. Christopherson, W. M., Collier, H. S.: Primary benign liver-cell tumors in infancy and childhood. Cancer *6*, 853–861 (1953)

26. Christopherson, W. M., Mays, E. T.: Liver tumors and contraceptive steroids. Experience with one hundred registry patients. J. Natl. Cancer Inst. *58*, 167–171 (1977)

27. Christopherson, W. M., Mays, E. T., Barrows, G. H.: Liver tumors in women on contraceptive steroids. Obstet. Gynecol. *48*, 221–223 (1975)

28. Christopherson, W. M., Mays, E. T., Barrows, G.: A clinicopathologic study of steroid-related tumors. Am. J. Surg. Pathol. *1*, 31–41 (1977)

29. Classen, M., Elster, K., Pesch, H. J., Demling, L.: Portal hypertension caused by partial nodular transformation of the liver. Gut *11*, 245–249 (1970)

30. Connolly, C., O'Brien, M. J.: Nodular transformation of the liver. Hum. Path. *8*, 350–352 (1977)

31. Contostavlos, D. L.: Benign hepatomas and oral contraceptives. Lancet *2*, 1200 (1973)

32. Cornish, P. G.: Liver cell adenoma. JAMA *235*, 249 (1976)

33. Davies, J. N. P.: Liver tumours and steroid hormones. Lancet *1*, 516 (1974)

34. Davis, J. B., Schenken, K. R., Zimmerman, O.: Massive hemoperitoneum from rupture of benign hepatocellular adenoma. Surgery *73*, 181–184 (1973)

35. Davis, M., Postmann, B., Searle, M., Wright, R., Williams, R.: Histological evidence of carcinoma in a hepatic tumour associated with oral contraceptives. Br. Med. J. *2*, 496–498 (1975)

36. Dick, A. P., Gresham, G. A.: Partial nodular transformation of the liver presenting with ascites. Gut *13*, 289–292 (1972)

37. Editorial: Oral contraceptives and cancer. Lancet *2*, 911 (1972)

38. Editorial: Liver tumours and steroid hormones. Lancet *2*, 1481–1482 (1973)

39. Editorial: Liver tumours and the pill. Br. Med. J. *2*, 3–4 (1974)

40. Editorial: Oral contraceptives and liver nodules. Lancet *1*, 843 (1976)

41. Edmonds, A. M., Hennigar, G. R., Crooks, R.: Galactosemia. Pediatrics *10*, 40–47 (1952)

42. Edmondson, H. A.: Tumors of the liver and Intrahepatic Bile Ducts. Atlas of Tumor Pathology, Sect. VII, Fasc. 25. Washington, D.C.: Armed Forces Inst. Pathol., 1958

43. Edmondson, H. A., Henderson, B. E., Benton, B.: Liver-cell adenomas associated with use of oral contraceptives. New Engl. J. Med. *294*, 470–472 (1976)

44. Edmondson, H. A., Reynolds, T. B., Henderson, B. E., Benton, B.: Regression of liver cell adenomas associated with oral contraceptives. Ann. Intern. Med. *86*, 180–182 (1977)

45. Everson, R. B., Fraumeni, J. F., Jr.: Familial glioblastoma with hepatic focal nodular hyperplasia. Cancer *38*, 310–313 (1976)

46. Everson, R. B., Museles, M., Henson, D. E., Grundy, G. W.: Focal nodular hyperplasia of the liver in a child with hemihypertrophy. J. Pediatr. *88*, 985–987 (1976)

47. Farber, E.: On the pathogenesis of experimental hepatocellular carcinoma. In: Hepatocellular Carcinoma. Okuda, K., Peters, R. L. (Eds.). New York: John Wiley and Sons, 1976, pp. 1–22

48. Farrell, G. C., Joshua, D. E., Uren, R. F., Baird, J. J., Perkins, K. W., Kronenberg, H.: Androgen-induced hepatoma. Lancet *1*, 430–432 (1975)

49. Fechner, R. E.: Benign hepatic lesions and orally administered contraceptives. A report of seven cases and a critical analysis of the literature. Hum. Pathol. *8*, 255–268 (1977)

50. Fechner, R. E., Roehm, J. O. F.: Angiographic and pathologic correlations of hepatic focal nodular hyperplasia. Am. J. Surg. Pathol. *1*, 217–224 (1977)

51. Fisher, A. W. F., Curry, B., Jacques, J.: Solitary liver nodules. Can. Med. Assoc. J. *112*, 1196–1200 (1975)
52. Galloway, S. J., Casarella, W. J., Lattes, R., Seaman, W. B.: Minimal deviation hepatoma. A new entity. Am. J. Roentgenol. *125*, 184–192 (1975)
53. Glassberg, A. B., Rosenbaum, E. H.: Oral contraceptives and malignant hepatoma. Lancet *1*, 479 (1976)
54. Goldfarb, S.: Sex hormones and hepatic neoplasia. Cancer Res. *36*, 2584–2588 (1976)
55. Goldstein, H. M., Neiman, H. L., Mena, E., Bookstein, J. J., Appelman, H. D.: Angiographic findings in benign liver cell tumors. Radiology *110*, 339–343 (1973)
56. Grabowski, M., Stenram, U., Bergqvist, A.: Focal nodular hyperplasia of the liver, benign hepatomas, oral contraceptives and other drugs affecting the liver. Acta Pathol. Microbiol. Scand. *83*, 615–622 (1975)
57. Guy, J. T., Auslander, M. O.: Androgenic steroids and hepatocellular carcinoma. Lancet *1*, 148 (1973)
58. Harris, M., Rash, R. M., Dymock, I. W.: Nodular non-cirrhotic liver associated with portal hypertension in a patient with rheumatoid arthritis. J. Clin. Pathol. *27*, 963–966 (1974)
59. Havrilla, T. R., Pepe, R. G., Alfidi, R. J., Haaga, J. R.: Benign hepatic tumors and cysts in women using contraceptive agents. Cleveland Clin. Q. *44*, 41–47 (1977)
60. Henderson, B. E., Benton, B., Edmondson, H. A.: Hepatocellular carcinoma and oral contraceptives. JAMA *236*, 560 (1976)
61. Henderson, J. T., Richmond, J., Sumerling, M. D.: Androgenic-anabolic steroid therapy and hepatocellular carcinoma. Lancet *1*, 934 (1973)
62. Henson, S. W., Gray, H. K., Dockerty, M. B.: Benign tumors of the liver. 1. Adenomas. Surg. Gynecol. Obstet. *103*, 23–30 (1956)
63. Hermann, R. E., David, T. E.: Spontaneous rupture of the liver caused by hepatomas. Surgery *74*, 715–719 (1973)
64. Holder, L. E., Gnarra, D. J., Lampkin, B. C., Nishiyama, H., Perkins, P.: Hepatoma associated with anabolic steroid therapy. Am. J. Roentgenol. *124*, 638–642 (1975)
65. Horvath, E., Kovacs, K., Ross, S. C.: Benign hepatoma in a young woman on contraceptive steroids. Lancet *1*, 357–358 (1974)
66. Howell, R. R., Stevenson, R. E., Ben-Menachem, Y., Phyliky, R. L., Berry, D. H.: Hepatic adenomata with type I glycogen storage disease. JAMA *236*, 1481–1484 (1976)
67. Irey, N. S., Norris, H. J.: Intimal vascular lesions associated with female reproductive steroids. Arch. Pathol. *96*, 227–234 (1973)
68. Irey, N. S., Manion, W. C., Taylor, H. B.: Vascular lesions in women taking oral contraceptives. Arch. Pathol. *89*, 1–8 (1970)
69. Ishak, K. G.: Primary hepatic tumors in childhood. In: Progress in Liver Diseases. Popper, H., Schaffner, F. (Eds.). New York: Grune and Stratton, 1976, pp. 636–667
70. Ishak, K. G., Rabin, L.: Benign tumors of the liver. Med. Clin. North Am. *59*, 995–1013 (1975)
71. Jhingran, A. K., Mukhopadhyay, A. K., Ajmani, S. K., Johnson, P. C.: Hepatic adenomas and focal nodular hyperplasia of the liver in young women on oral contraceptives. Case reports. J. Nucl. Med. *18*, 263–266 (1977)
72. Johnson, F. L.: Androgenic-anabolic steroids and hepatocellular carcinoma. In: Hepatocellular Carcinoma. Okuda, K., Peters, R. L. (Eds.). New York: John Wiley and Sons, 1976, pp. 95–103
73. Johnson, F. L., Feagler, J. R., Lerner, K. G., Majerus, P. W., Siegel, M., Hartmann, J. R., Thomas, E. D.: Association of androgenic-anabolic steroid therapy with development of hepatocellular carcinoma. Lancet *2*, 1273–1276 (1972)
74. Kalra, T. M. S., Mangla, J. C., DePapp, E. W.: Benign hepatic tumors and oral contraceptive pills. Am. J. Med. *61*, 871–877 (1976)
75. Kay, C. R.: Oral contraceptives and liver tumours. Lancet *2*, 127 (1975)

76. Kay, S., Schatzki, P. F.: Ultrastructure of a benign liver cell adenoma. Cancer 28, 755–762 (1971)
77. Kelso, D. R.: Benign hepatomas and oral contraceptives. Lancet 1, 315–316 (1974)
78. Kew, M. C., Van Coller, B., Prowse, C. M., Skikne, B., Wolfsdorf, J. I., Isdale, J., Krawitz, S., Altman, H., Levin, S. E., Bothwell, T. H.: Occurrence of primary hepatocellular cancer and peliosis hepatis arter treatment with androgenic steroids. S. Afr. Med. J. 50, 1233–1237 (1976)
79. Klatskin, G.: Hepatic tumors. Possible relationship to use of oral contraceptives. Gastroenterology 73, 386–394 (1977)
80. Knapp, W. A., Ruebner, B. H.: Hepatomas and oral contraceptives. Lancet 1, 270–271 (1974)
81. Knowles, D. M., Wolff, M.: Focal nodular hyperplasia of the liver. A clinicopathologic study and review of the literature. Hum. Pathol. 7, 533–545 (1976)
82. Knowles, D. M., Kaye, G. I., Godman, G. C.: Nodular regenerative hyperplasia of the liver. Gastroenterology 69, 746–751 (1975)
83. Koka, M., Stejskal, R., Wagner, B., Rao, J. S., McDonnell, R. G.: Pathologic effects of Ovulen (R) and Enovid-E (R) on beagle dogs after 7 years of treatment. XI Intern. Congr., Intern. Acad. Pathol., October 17–23. Washington, D.C. (Abstract), 1976
84. Lansing, P. B., McQuitty, J. T., Bradburn, D. M.: Benign liver tumors: What is their relationship to oral contraceptives. Am. Surg. 42, 744–760 (1976)
85. Leevy, C. M., Popper, H., Sherlock, S.: Diseases of the Liver and Biliary Tract, Standardization of Nomenclature, Diagnostic Criteria, and Diagnostic Methodology. Fogarty International Center Proceedings No. 22. Washington, D.C.: U.S. Government Printing Office 1976, pp. 1–212
86. Lesna, M., Spencer, I., Wolker, W.: Liver nodules and androgens. Lancet 1, 1124 (1976)
87. Lingeman, C. H.: Evaluating carcinogenicity of oral contraceptives. JAMA 236, 1690 (1976)
88. Lurie, B., Novis, B., Bank, S., Silver, W., Botha, J. B. C., Marks, I. N.: CRST syndrome and nodular transformation of the liver. Gastroenterology 64, 457–461 (1973)
89. Maillard, J. N., Potet, F., Benhamou, J. P.: Transformation nodulaire partielle du foie avec hypertension portale. Presse Med. 75, 2799–2802 (1967)
90. Mahboubi, E., Shubik, P.: Benign liver cell adenomas in women using oral contraceptives. Cancer Lett. 1, 331–338 (1976)
91. Malt, R. A., Hershberg, R. A., Miller, W. L.: Experience with benign tumors of the liver. Surg. Gynecol. Obstet. 130, 285–291 (1970)
92. Mays, E. T.: Hepatocellular carcinoma and oral contraceptives. JAMA 236, 560 (1976)
93. Mays, E. T., Christopherson, W. H., Barrows, G. H.: Focal nodular hyperplasia of the liver. Possible relationship to oral contraceptives. Am. J. Clin. Pathol. 61, 735–746 (1974)
94. Mays, E. T., Christopherson, W. M., Mahr, M. M., Williams, H. C.: Hepatic changes in young women ingesting contraceptive steroids: hepatic hemorrhage and primary hepatic tumors. JAMA 235, 730–732 (1976)
95. McAvoy, J. M., Tompkins, R. K., Longmire, W. P., Jr.: Benign hepatic tumors and their association with oral contraceptives. Arch. Surg. 111, 761–767 (1976)
96. McKinney, G. R., Weikel, J. H., Jr., Webb, W. K., Dick, R. G.: Use of the life-table technique to estimate effects of certain steroids on probability of tumor formation in a long-term study in rats. Toxicol. Appl. Pharmacol. 12, 68–79 (1968)
97. McLoughlin, M. J., Gilday, D. L.: Angiography and colloid scanning of benign mass lesions of the liver. Clin. Radiol. 23, 377–391 (1973)
98. McLoughlin, M. J., Colapinto, R. F., Gilday, D. L., Hobbs, B. B., Korobkin, M. T., McDonald, P., Phillips, M. J.: Focal nodular hyperplasia of the liver. Angiography and radioisotope scanning. Radiology 107, 257–263 (1973)
99. Meadows, A. T., Naiman, J. L., Valdes-Dapena, M.: Hepatoma associated with androgen therapy for aplastic anemia. J. Pediatr. 84, 108–110 (1974)

100. Meyer, P., Livolsi, V. A., Cornog, J. L.: Hepatoblastoma associated with an oral contraceptive. Lancet 2, 1387 (1974)
101. Minow, R. A., Tompkins, R. K., Gitnick, G. L.: Diarrhea syndrome in hepatic adenoma. Am. J. Dig. Dis. 20, 182–186 (1975)
102. Model, D. G., Fox, J. A., Jones, R. W.: Multiple hepatic adenomas associated with an oral contraceptive. Lancet 1, 865 (1975)
103. Mokrohisky, S. T., Ambruso, D. R., Hathaway, W. E.: Fulminant hepatic neoplasia after androgen therapy. New Engl. J. Med. 296, 1411–1412 (1977)
104. Morley, J. E., Myers, J. B., Sack, F. S., Kalk, F., Epstein, E. E., Lannon, J.: Enlargement of cavernous haemangioma associated with exogenous administration of oestrogens. S. Afr. Med. J. 1, 695–697 (1974)
105. Morton, R. F., Hebel, J. R.: Liver-cell adenomas and oral contraceptives. New Engl. J. Med. 295, 52 (1976)
106. Motsay, G. J., Gamble, W. G.: Clinical experience with hepatic adenomas. Surg. Gynecol. Obstet. 134, 415–418 (1972)
107. Mowat, A. P., Gutjahr, P., Portmann, B., Dawson, J. L., Williams, R.: Focal nodular hyperplasia of the liver. A rational approach to treatment. Gut 17, 492–494 (1976)
108. Mulvihill, J. J., Ridolfi, R. L., Schultz, F. R., Borzy, M. S., Haughton, P. B. T.: Hepatic adenoma in Fanconi anemia treated with oxymetholone. J. Pediatr. 87, 122–124 (1975)
109. Nadell, J., Kosek, J.: Peliosis hepatis. Twelve cases associated with oral androgen therapy. Arch. Pathol. Lab. Med. 101, 405–410 (1977)
110. Nikaidoh, H., Boggs, J., Swenson, O.: Liver tumors in infants and children. Clinical and pathological analysis of 22 cases. Arch. Surg. 101, 245–257 (1970)
111. Nissen, E. D., Kent, D. R.: Liver tumors and oral contraceptives. Obstet. Gynecol. 46, 460–467 (1975)
112. Oral Contraceptives and Health. An Interim Report from the Oral Contraception Study of the Royal College of General Practitioners. New York: Pitman Publishing Corporation, 1974, pp. 1–100
113. Osterholzer, H. O., Grillo, D., Kruger, P. S., Dunnihoo, D. R.: The effect of oral contraceptive steroids on branches of the uterine artery. Obstet. Gynecol. 49, 227–232 (1977)
114. O'Sullivan, J. P.: Oral contraceptives and liver tumours. Proc. R. Soc. Med. 69, 351–353 (1976)
115. O'Sullivan, J. P., Rosswick, R. P.: Oral contraceptives and malignant hepatic tumors. Lancet 1, 1124–1125 (1976)
116. O'Sullivan, J. P., Wilding, R. P.: Liver hamartomas in patients on oral contraceptives. Br. Med. J. 2, 7–10 (1974)
117. Phillips, M. J., Langer, B., Stone, R., Fisher, M. M., Ritchie, S.: Benign liver cell tumors. Classification and ultrastructural pathology. Cancer 32, 463–470 (1973)
118. Pollice, L.: Primary hepatic tumors in infancy and childhood. Am. J. Clin. Pathol. 60, 512–521 (1973)
119. Port, R. B., Patasnick, J. P., Ranniger, K.: Angiographic demonstration of hepatoma in association with Fanconi's anemia. Am. J. Roentgenol. 113, 82–83 (1971)
120. Pryor, A. G., Cohen, R. J., Goldman, R. L.: Hepatocellular carcinoma in a woman on long-term oral contraceptives. Cancer 40, 884–888 (1977)
121. Recant, L., Lacey, P.: Fanconi's anemia and hepatic cirrhosis. Clinicopathologic conference. Am. J. Med. 39, 464–475 (1965)
122. Reisman, T., Levi, J. U., Zeppa, R., Clark, R., Morton, R., Schiff, E. R.: Noncirrhotic portal hypertension in Felty's syndrome. Am. J. Dig. Dis. 22, 145–148 (1977)
123. Rinehart, W., Felt, J. C.: Debate on oral contraceptives and neoplasia continues; answers remain elusive. Population Reports, Series A, Number 4, 69–104 (1977)
124. Rinehart, W., Ravenholt, R. T.: U.S. Morbidity and mortality trends relative to oral contraceptive use, 1955–1975, and Danish morbidity trends, 1953–1972. Population Reports, Series A, Number 4, 105–142 (1977)

125. Rooks, J. B., Ory, H. W., Ishak, K. G., Strauss, L. T., Greenspan, J. R., Tyler, C. W.: Association of hepatocellular adenoma and oral contraception. A case controlled study (In preparation)

126. Ross, D., Pina, J., Mirza, M., Galvan, A., Ponce, L.: Regression of focal nodular hyperplasia after discontinuation of oral contraceptives. Ann. Intern. Med. *85*, 203—204 (1976)

127. Sale, G. E., Lerner, K. G.: Multiple tumors after androgen therapy. Arch. Pathol. Lab. Med. *101*, 600—603 (1977)

128. Sarna, G., Tomasulo, P., Lotz, M. J., Bubinak, J. F., Shulman, N. R.: Multiple neoplasms in two siblings with a variant form of Fanconi's anemia. Cancer *36*, 1029—1033 (1975)

129. Schardein, J. L., Kaump, D. H., Woosley, E. T., Jellema, M. M.: Long-term toxicologic and tumorigenesis studies on an oral contraceptive agent in albino rats. Toxicol. Appl. Pharmacol. *16*, 10—23 (1970)

130. Sherlock, S., Feldman, C. A., Moran, B., Scheuer, P. J.: Partial nodular transformation of the liver with portal hypertension. Am. J. Med. *40*, 195—203 (1966)

131. Sorenson, T. I. A., Baden, H.: Benign hepatocellular tumours. Scand. J. Gastroenterol. *10*, 113—119 (1975)

132. Squire, R. A., Levitt, M. H.: Report of a workshop on classification of specific hepatocellular lesions in rats. Cancer Res. *35*, 3214—3223 (1975)

133. Stauffer, J. Q., Hill, R. B.: Systemic contraceptives and liver tumors. Ann. Intern. Med. *85*, 122—123 (1976)

134. Stauffer, J. Q., Lapinski, M. W., Honold, D. J., Myers, J. K.: Focal nodular hyperplasia of the liver and intrahepatic hemorrhage in young women on oral contraceptives. Ann. Intern. Med. *83*, 301—306 (1975)

135. Steiner, P. E.: Nodular regenerative hyperplasia of the liver. Am. J. Pathol. *35*, 943—953 (1959)

136. Steinherz, P. B., Canale, V. C., Miller, D. R.: Hepatocellular carcinoma, transfusion-induced hemochromatosis and congenital hypoplastic anemia (Blackfan-Diamond syndrome). Am. J. Med. *60*, 1032—1035 (1976)

137. Stenwig, A. E., Solgaard, T.: Recurrent benign hepatoma associated with an oral contraceptive. A case report. Virchows Arch. *367*, 337—343 (1975)

138. Sweeney, E. C. and Evans, D. J.: Liver lesions and androgenic steroid therapy. Lancet *2*, 1042 (1975)

139. Sweeney, E. C., Evans, D. J.: Hepatic lesions in patients treated with synthetic anabolic steroids. J. Clin. Pathol. *29*, 626—633 (1976)

140. Teng, C. T., Daeschner, C. W., Jr., Singleton, E. B., Rosenberg, H. S., Cole, V. S., Hills, L. L., Brennan, J. C.: Liver disease and osteoporosis in children. I. Clinical observations. J. Pediatr. *59*, 684—702 (1961)

141. Thalassinos, N. C., Lymberatos, C., Hadjioannou, J., Gardikas, C.: Liver-cell carcinoma after long-term oestrogen-like drugs. Lancet *1*, 270 (1974)

142. Thomas, P. A., McCusker, J. J., Merrigan, E. H., Conte, N. F.: Lobar cirrhosis with nodular hyperplasia (hamartoma) of the liver treated by left hepatic lobectomy. Am. J. Surg. *112*, 831—834 (1966)

143. Thorkild, I. A., Sorensen, A., Almersjo, O.: Focal nodular hyperplasia of the liver. Five cases. Scand. J. Gastroenterol. *11*, 97—101 (1976)

144. Tigano, F., Ferlazzo, B., Barrile, A.: Oral contraceptives and malignant hepatoma. Lancet *2*, 196 (1976)

145. Tountas, C., Paraskevas, G., Deligeorgi, H.: Benign hepatoma and oral contraceptives. Lancet *1*, 1351—1352 (1974)

146. Tsou, K. C., Ledis, S., McCoy, M. G.: 5'nucleotide phosphodiesterase isoenzyme pattern in the serum of human hepatoma. Cancer Res. *33*, 2215—2217 (1973)

147. Tyrer, L. B.: Liver-cell adenomas and oral contraceptives. New Engl. J. Med. *295*, 51—52 (1976)

148. Uszler, J. M., Swanson, L. A.: Focal nodular hyperplasia of the liver. Case report. J. Nucl. Med. *16*, 831–832 (1975)
149. Vessey, M. P., Kay, C. R., Baldwin, J. A., Clarke, J. A., MacLeod, J. B.: Oral contraceptives and benign liver tumours. Br. Med. J. *1*, 1064–1065 (1977)
150. Wazeter, F. X., Geil, R. G., Cookson, K. M., Berliner, V. R., Lamar, J. K.: Seven-year progress report on long-term oral contraceptive studies in female dogs and monkeys (Abstract). Toxicol. Appl. Pharmacol. *37*, 178 (1976)
151. Whelan, T. J., Baugh, J. H., Chandor, S.: Focal nodular hyperplasia of the liver. Ann. Surg. *177*, 150–158 (1973)
152. Wilens, G.: Adenoma of the liver. Am. J. Dis. Child. *55*, 792–797 (1928)
153. Winckler, K., Poulsen, H.: Liver disease with periportal sinusoidal dilatation. A possible complication to contraceptive steroids. Scand. J. Gastroenterol. *10*, 699–704 (1975)
154. World Health Organzation. Report of the Meeting of Investigators on the Histological Classification of Tumors of the Liver, Biliary Tract and Pancreas. Switzerland, Nov. 24–28, 1975, pp. 1–22, Geneva
155. Ziegenfuss, J., Carabasi, R.: Androgens and hepatocellular carcinoma. Lancet *1*, 262 (1973)

Mammary Neoplasia in Animals: Pathologic Aspects and the Effects of Contraceptive Steroids[1]

H. W. Casey, R. C. Giles, and R. P. Kwapien[2]

Introduction

The incidence of spontaneous tumors of the mammary gland varies greatly among the different mammalian species. Large domesticated animals have a very low frequency of the disease. Even though the cow has enormous mammary gland development and cows numbering in the millions are observed to an old age, less than 50 cases have been reported in the literature. Similarly, mammary tumors are equally rare in sheep, horses, pigs, and goats. In contrast, the incidence of mammary tumors in the dog exceeds that of women by a factor of 3 to 4, and the disease is common in the cat. Rats and mice have a high incidence of mammary tumors; however, they are less frequent in other species of small laboratory animals. Mammary neoplasms are apparently rare in the nonhuman primate, but interest in the disease in these animals remains high as they have a menstrual cycle comparable to women. This paper reviews some major aspects of spontaneous mammary tumors in mice, rats, cats, dogs, and nonhuman primates. Emphasis has been placed on the pathologic aspects of the neoplasms and the use of these species in the carcinogenic testing of contraceptive steroids. The literature contains a large number of excellent publications on mammary neoplasia in animals; only selected articles are cited. The reader is especially referred to the comprehensive review by HAMILTON published in 1974 [32] and the review by STEWART published in 1976 [68] on the comparative pathology of animal neoplasia.

Mice

The incidence of mammary tumors in the laboratory mouse varies remarkably among the different strains. In strains with high incidence, nearly 100% of the females may develop the disease, while in the strains with low incidence the frequency of the disease is less than 5%. The C3H strain of mice has been used repeatedly in the study of mammary neoplasia, as 80%–90% of breeder females develop mammary tumors before 1 year of age. In contrast, the C57BL mouse seldom develops mammary tumors even when maintained to old age [58].

1 Partially supported by NIH/NICHD contract No. NO1-HD-2-2729, from the Contraceptive Evaluation Branch, National Institute of Child Health and Human Development, National Institutes of Health, Public Health Service, U.S. Department of Health, Education and Welfare, Bethesda, MD. 20014.

2 The opinions or assertions contained herein are the private views of the authors and are not to be construed as official or as reflecting the views of the Department of the Army, of the Air Force, or of Defense.

The vast majority of mammary tumors occur in strains of mice that are genetically susceptible to the mouse mammary tumor virus (MMTV) [42, 50, 51, 52]. This virus, originally detected in the milk by BITTNER in 1936, has been extensively studied in the mouse as a model of viral carcinogenesis. The agent is an RNA virus that multiplies in the cytoplasm and generally appears as a type B particle. It is now recognized that a number of variants of the MMTV exist. Some variants may be transmitted in certain strains of mice by the germ cells of both the male and female, and both exogenous and endogenous forms of the virus are known to exist [50, 52, 58]. Despite the known existence of different variants, even within the same strain of mice, most strains of mice with a high incidence of mammary tumors carry large amounts of infective virus. Conversely, in strains of mice in which the infective virus cannot be demonstrated by routine techniques, it should not be assumed that the mouse is free of all variant forms of the virus.

The classification of mammary tumors of the mouse is relatively standardized and is primarily based on the excellent descriptions and terminology published by DUNN in 1959 [21]. The vast majority of mouse mammary tumors develop from the luminal or secretory cell of acinar origin. It is recognized that the histologic appearance of mammary neoplasms in the mouse cannot be correlated with their metastatic potential. As a result, nearly all mouse mammary tumors are considered to be carcinomas. Two precancerous lesions are recognized in the mouse, the hyperplastic alveolar nodule (HAN) and the pregnancy-responsive plaque. In addition to carcinomas, occasional sarcomas and carcinosarcomas occur in the mouse mammary gland. The vast majority of mouse mammary tumors can be classified as either adenocarcinomas of types A, B, C, or adenoacanthomas. The type A adenocarcinoma is a well-differentiated neoplasm composed of uniform acini or small tubules lined by a single layer of epithelium that may show secretory activity (Figs. 1 and 2). The tumor is locally invasive and even though highly differentiated may metastasize via the blood stream to the lungs. Type B adenocarcinomas are composed of the same type acinar cell as seen in type A but show a marked variation in their patterns, with the cells arranged in solid lobules, cords, or

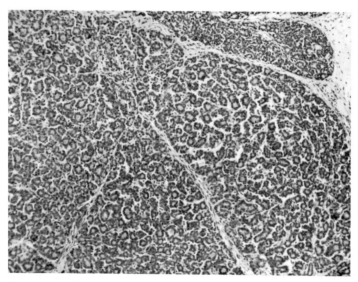

Fig. 1. Type A adenocarcinoma, mouse. AFIP Neg. No. 77-5082, H & E × 100

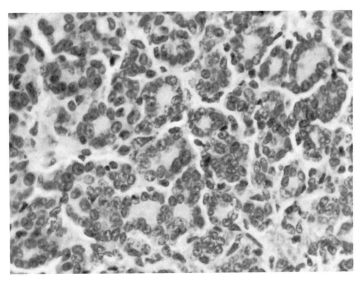

Fig. 2. Type A adenocarcinoma illustrating well-differentiated acinar formations, mouse. AFIP Neg. No. 77-5089, H & E, × 485

papillary and tubular configurations with large cystic areas (Figs. 3 and 4). Type A and B adenocarcinoma patterns may both appear within the same mammary tumor. The A and B type adenocarcinomas are generally associated with virus-induced tumors and are seen in mice at a relatively young age [21, 71]. The type C adenocarcinoma is an infrequent neoplasm seen in older mice and is generally not considered to be of viral origin [21]. This neoplasm is

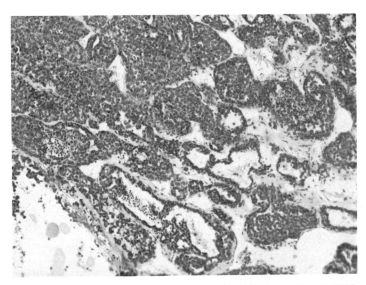

Fig. 3. Type B adenocarcinoma with solid and glandular areas, mouse. AFIP Neg. No. 77-5282, H & E, × 100

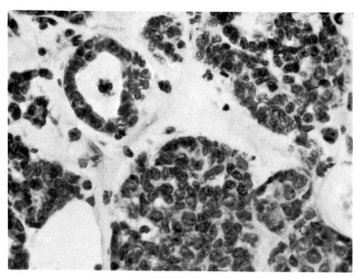

Fig. 4. Higher magnification of Type B adenocarcinoma illustrated in Figure 3. AFIP Neg. No. 77-5292, H & E, × 485

composed of acini and tubules that may assume an organoid appearance. The acinar and tubular structures are generally lined by a single layer of epithelial cells and are surrounded by characteristically loose and edematous stroma thought to be of myoepithelial cell origin (Figs. 5 and 6). This stroma may contain scattered collagen fibers, a feature which has led some authors to term this neoplasm a fibroadenoma [71]. Adenoacanthomas also occur in older mice and are generally not considered to be of viral origin. Some authors [71] believe this

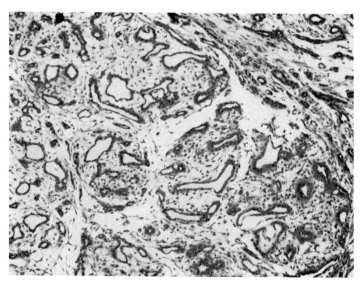

Fig. 5. Type C adenocarcinoma, mouse. AFIP Neg. No. 77-5505, H & E, × 100

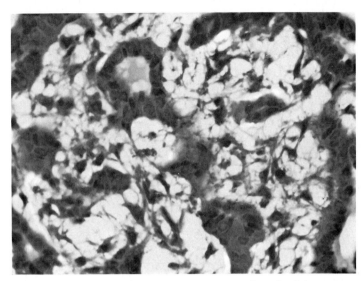

Fig. 6. Type C adenocarcinoma illustrating loose edematous tissue surrounding glandular components, mouse. AFIP Neg. No. 77-5335, H & E, × 485

lesion arises from ducts as the result of hormonal stimulation. DUNN considered the tumor a variant of adenocarcinoma since glandular elements of the A and B type may form up to 75% of the tumor (Figs. 7 and 8). The squamous component of the tumor is considered an integral part of the lesion rather than a metaplastic change as this component also appears in metastatic sites [21]. Molluscoid and organoid variants of this tumor occur [21]. In addition to the carcinomas described by DUNN [21], VAN NIE and DUX [72] have described a pale-cell

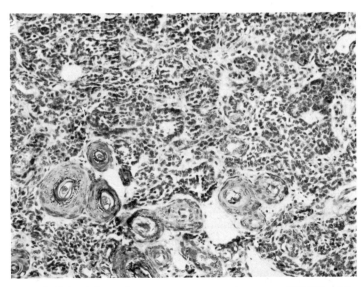

Fig. 7. Adenoacanthoma composed of glandular and squamous components, mouse. AFIP Neg. No. 77-5422, H & E, × 100

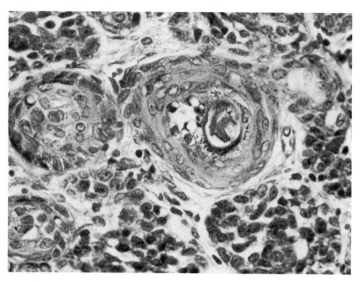

Fig. 8. Higher magnification of adenoacanthoma in Figure 7 illustrating squamous cells and keratin formation. AFIP Neg. No. 77-5091, H & E, × 485

carcinoma, type P, that develops in the GR mouse from preneoplastic pregnancy-responsive plaques [27]. This tumor is composed of large cells with abundant cytoplasm and pale oval nuclei. The cells are generally arranged in solid islands with a smaller, darker cell at the periphery of the islands.

Mouse mammary tumors are generally considered to be hormone independent once they develop. Estrogens and the pituitary hormone prolactin play a particularly important role in the development of precancerous lesions and subsequent tumor development [58, 76].

The effects of contraceptive steroids on the development of mammary tumors in mice have not been entirely clarified despite a large number of reported studies. This subject was reviewed in detail by an international committee in 1974 [43]. Most studies were not conducted in agreement with a standard protocol; a variety of strains, doses, and routes of administration were used and, thus, it is difficult to compare individual studies. In general, most studies indicated that the estrogenic compounds used alone or in combination with a progestin increased the frequency of mammary tumors in mice. This effect is generally more consistent with higher doses and more pronounced in male mice. Studies with the 17 α-hydroxyprogesterone derivatives, chlormadinone acetate, and megestrol acetate [10], all without estrogen, did not have an effect on the frequency of mammary tumors. When these drugs were administered with estrogen, they produced mammary tumors in male mice. The 19-nortestosterone derivatives, ethynodiol diacetate, norethisterone, norethynodrel, and nor-gestrel, administered without estrogen, had no effect on the frequency of mammary tumors in female mice. In one study, the incidence of mammary tumors in castrated male mice was increased by norethynodrel. In some studies, combination drugs, 19-nortestosterone with estrogen, increased the number of mammary tumors in female mice and frequently increased the number of mammary tumors in male mice. Generally, in studies that demonstrated an increase in the number of mammary tumors, the effect was most obvious with high doses, i.e., 50—400 times the recommended human dose.

Little attention has been paid to the morphologic aspects of the tumors seen in mice administered contraceptive steroids and in most studies the tumors were simply described as carcinomas.

Rats

Mammary tumors are common in all strains of laboratory rats. Similarly to the mouse, this species has been used extensively in the study of experimental mammary carcinogenesis. For a comprehensive reference on the pathology of the mammary tumor of the rat, the reader is referred to the review by YOUNG and HALLOWES published in 1973 [77]. The frequency of rat mammary tumors may vary greatly, not only among different strains, but — more important — in animals of the same strain maintained in different laboratories. Even with the same strain maintained in the same laboratory, reports of the frequency of the disease may vary greatly in studies performed at different times [67]. In most studies, the number of rats developing mammary tumors varies from 10% to 60%; however, percentages of less than 10 to over 90 have frequently been reported [67]. Occasionally, mammary tumors develop in rats less than 1 year old, but most occur between 1 and 2 years of age and additional tumors continue to develop throughout life [22]. The development of multiple tumors in an individual rat is not uncommon.

The vast majority of the spontaneous mammary tumors in rats are benign (80%—90%) and are generally classified histologically as fibroadenomas. Despite this high incidence of histologically benign tumors, a variety of histologic types of carcinomas occur. In 1973, the International Agency for Research on Cancer (IARC) [77] published a classification of rat mammary tumors in an effort to standardize nomenclature for tumors of laboratory animals. The IARC classification recognized lobular hyperplasia (adenosis) as a proliferative non-neoplastic lesion consisting of normal acini arranged in a lobular pattern substantially larger than adjacent lobules. The classification lists three benign tumors: adenomas, fibroadenomas, and fibromas. Histologically, adenomas are composed of acini, lined by a single layer of secretory epithelium, containing a normal complement of myoepithelial cells (Figs. 9 and 10). The adenomas generally maintain a lobular pattern, although distortion of some lobules may be present. In our experience solitary adenomas are uncommon, but adenomatous hyperplasia of lobules is frequently observed in association with fibroadenomatous tumors. Both the intracanalicular and pericanalicular types of fibroadenoma occur, and the latter type is by far the most common (Figs. 11 and 12). The amount of fibrous tissue in the fibroadenoma may vary tremendously. Some authors have used the term "adenofibroma" to describe tumors with a large complement of adenomatous structures in relation to stroma. Likewise, tumors composed almost entirely of fibrous tissue have been termed "fibromas" a designation recognized in the IARC classification. The epithelial component of the fibroadenoma is composed of acini lined by a single layer of epithelium that may or may not show secretory activity. Cellular atypia is not a feature of the fibroadenoma, but nuclei that are dense and atrophic in appearance are frequently observed and represent degenerative changes. Intracanalicular fibroadenomas are relatively rare and must be distinguished from carcinomas that have a lobular canalicular pattern. Although fibroadenomas in the rat do not metastasize, they continue to grow and occasionally become larger than the animal.

Carcinomas of the rat exhibit a variety of histologic patterns. The IARC classification lists adeno-, papillary, anaplastic, cribriform, comedo, and squamous carcinomas as occurring in the rat. The diagnosis of carcinomas in this species is generally based on histologic criteria

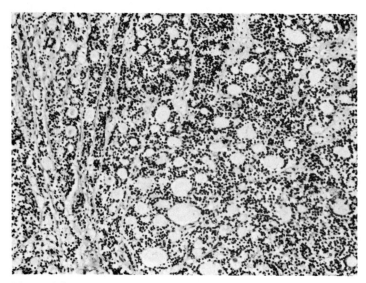

Fig. 9. Adenoma, rat. AFIP Neg. No. 77-5423, H & E, × 100

rather than proven metastatic potential. Probably less than 10% of tumors diagnosed as carcinomas metastasize; however, criteria have not been established to distinguish metastasizing and nonmetastasizing tumors with any consistency. Carcinomas that metastasize usually go to the lungs via the blood stream. The principal histologic features of carcinoma in the rat involve alteration in the arrangement of the cells coupled with varying degrees of

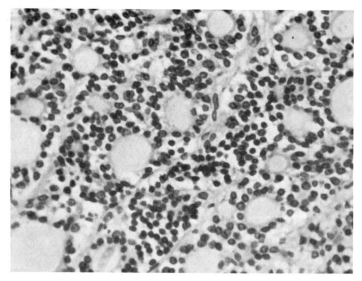

Fig. 10. Higher magnification of adenoma in Figure 9 illustrating acini with secretory activities. AFIP Neg. No. 77-5086, H & E, × 485

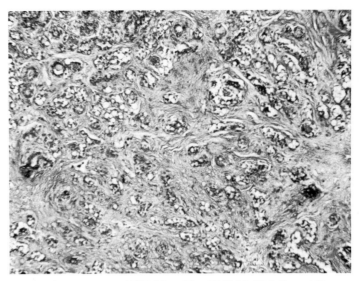

Fig. 11. Fibroadenoma, pericanalicular type, rat. AFIP Neg. No. 77-5286, H & E, × 100

cellular anaplasia. Many types of carcinoma still retain a semblance of lobular patterns (Figs. 13). Piling up of cells in tubular and acinar structures is a very common feature. Most carcinoma cells are larger than their normal counterpart and their nuclei frequently contain dense chromatin with prominent nucleoli. Mitotic figures are usually present in moderate to high numbers. Despite marked alteration in the morphology, secretory activity is present in

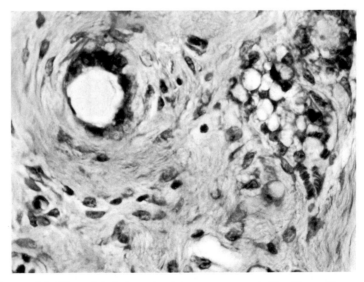

Fig. 12. Fibroadenoma illustrated in Figure 11. Acinar structures are surrounded by fibrous tissue. Epithelial cells show pyknotic nuclei and cytoplasmic vacuoles. AFIP Neg. No. 77-5289, H & E, × 485

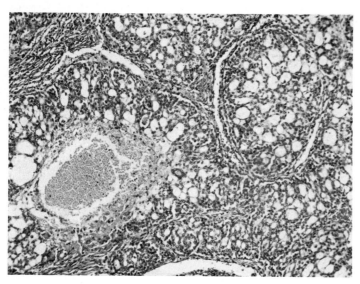

Fig. 13. Adenocarcinoma, cribriform-comedo type, rat. AFIP Neg. No. 77-5285, H & E, × 100

many carcinomas. In our experience, the most common forms of carcinoma are adeno- and cribriform types (Figs. 13–16). Comedo patterns are frequently observed in some cribriform carcinomas (Fig. 13). Sarcomas of the rat mammary gland are rare but occasionally occur in older animals, as do carcinosarcomas. Fibrosarcomas are the most common, and their possible development from malignant transformation of fibroadenomas has been suggested [77].

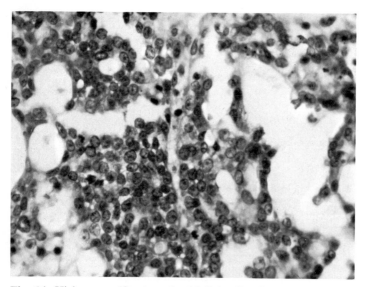

Fig. 14. Higher magnification of epithelial cells of the cribriform adenocarcinoma illustrated in Figure 13. AFIP Neg. No. 77-5290, H & E, × 485

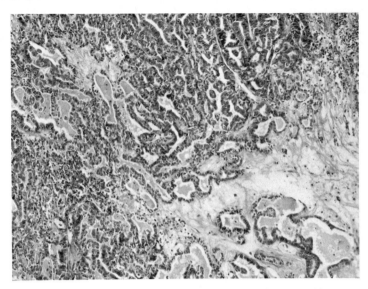

Fig. 15. Invasive tubular adenocarcinoma, rat. AFIP Neg. No. 77-5503, H & E, × 100

The administration of chemical carcinogens has been shown to increase the frequency and reduce the time of appearance of mammary tumors in rats [40, 41, 78]. This model for producing mammary tumors in the rat has been refined and has been used extensively in the study of mammary neoplasia. Most investigators use the carcinogen dimethylbenz[a]anthracene (DMBA), administered in a single dose of 20–50 mg at approximately 50 days of age. Mammary tumors subsequently develop in 75%–100% of female animals in 3–4 months.

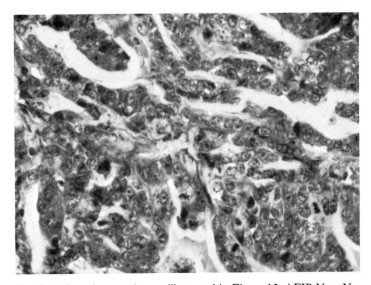

Fig. 16. Large anaplastic cells of tubular adenocarcinoma illustrated in Figure 15. AFIP Neg. No. 77-5291, H & E, × 485

Histologically, chemically induced mammary tumors display more anaplastic features than the naturally occurring tumors and are classified as carcinomas although metastasis is seldom observed [78].

The development of mammary tumors in the rat is dependent on ovarian, adrenal, and pituitary functions. Ovariectomy prior to 3 months of age markedly reduces the frequency of occurrence, and ovariectomy combined with adrenalectomy completely suppresses tumor development [22]. Carcinogen-induced mammary tumors in the rat are hormone dependent, as ovariectomy following development induces regressive changes. These regressive changes can be reversed in most tumors by the administration of estrogen; however, the administration of progesterone does not alter the regressive state. More recent work [6, 66] has shown that chemically induced mammary tumors in the Sprague-Dawley rat are estrogen and prolactin dependent and that the primary effect of estrogen is probably via the pituitary gland and prolactin.

The administration of exogenous estrogenic compounds to rats generally results in increased numbers of mammary tumors, particularly in male rats. This effect may be dependent on the dose administered, since it has not been observed in all studies [43]. Most reports describing an increase in mammary tumors in rats following the administration of contraceptive steroids were from studies in which progestin/estrogen combinations were used [10, 43]. Like the studies performed in mice, the protocols for the carcinogenic testing of contraceptive steroid drugs have not been standardized as to strain of rat, dosage, and route of administration. Studies have not reported an increase in mammary tumors in rats administered 17 α-hydroxyprogesterone with or without estrogen. Studies using 19-nortestosterone derivatives have shown that these drugs do not increase the frequency of mammary tumors when administered without estrogens. When norethynodrel or norethisterone acetate were given in combination with estrogen, some studies have shown an increase in mammary tumors in female rats. When the 19-nortestosterone drugs were administered to male rats, an increase in mammary tumors was seen; however, this effect has been observed most consistently when the drugs have been administered in combination with estrogens. For a review of the individual studies concerning the effects of these drugs on the rat mammary gland, readers should consult the IARC Monograph published in 1974 [43].

Detailed studies on the pathology of mammary neoplasms observed in rats administered the various contraceptive steroidal drugs are lacking and no attempts have been made to compare in detail the histology of these tumors, other than benign versus malignant, with spontaneous neoplasms.

Cats

The incidence of mammary tumors in cats exceeds that of all domestic animals other than the dog. Studies conducted in California on a population at risk found an annual incidence of 25.4 per 100,000 female cats [18]. Most of the literature on the disease has been directed toward the highly malignant nature of the neoplasms, as 80%—90% of all mammary tumors in the cat metastasize. A general review of this disease in cats was recently published by HAYES [35]. Mammary tumors have been reported in cats from 1 to 20 years of age [75]. The peak age is generally considered to be from 11 to 12 years [32]. The vast majority of feline mammary tumors develop from the secretory or luminal epithelial cells; however, rare mixed tumors have been reported. Most investigators [13, 34, 62, 75] have classified feline mammary tumors as adenomas, papillomas (Fig. 17), papillary and tubular adenocarcinomas (Figs. 18

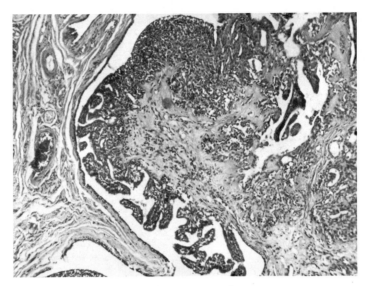

Fig. 17. Duct papilloma, cat. AFIP Neg. No. 77-5081, H & E, × 100

and 19) and solid carcinomas (Fig. 20). Many carcinomas may exhibit both solid and glandular areas. Rare mucoid carcinomas have also been seen in the cat [75]. Feline carcinomas readily metastasize to the lung, which may ultimately result in disseminated metastatic disease. WEIJER et al. [75] studied 179 feline carcinomas and reported that 151 cats died or were killed because of either metastatic or recurrent disease within 1 year of diagnosis.

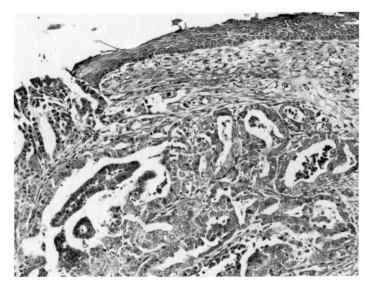

Fig. 18. Invasive tubular papillary adenocarcinoma with ulceration of the overlying epidermis, cat. AFIP Neg. No. 77-2686, H & E, × 120

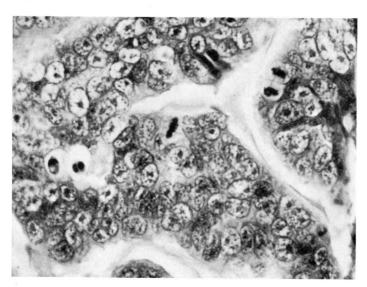

Fig. 19. Highly anaplastic cells of the papillary tubular adenocarcinoma illustrated in Figure 18. AFIP Neg. No. 77-2694, H & E, × 675

A proliferative non-neoplastic disease, feline mammary hyperplasia [1], has recently been reported in young cats. This lesion probably represents the entities previously described as fibroadenoma [34] or total fibromatoid change [33]. The lesion occurs primarily in young cats, may involve one or all glands, and may be due to hormonal aberrations.
Essentially no information is available on the etiologic aspects of the disease in cats. Limited studies indicate that hormones may play a role in the development of the disease, but good

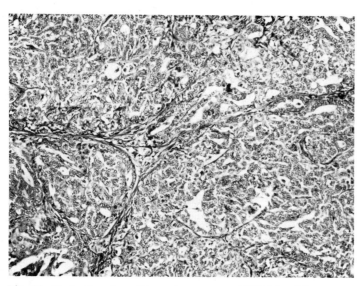

Fig. 20. Predominantly solid carcinoma, cat. AFIP Neg. No. 77-5502, H & E, × 50

experimental data are lacking. DORN et al. [18] presented data indicating that the risk of developing mammary cancer is 7 times greater in intact females than in ovariectomized animals. Other authors indicate that ovariectomized animals have a lower incidence of the disease (see review by HAYES [35]). Viruslike particles, C type, have been demonstrated ultrastructurally in feline mammary tumors [23]. The significance of these findings is unknown, as the feline leukemia virus, a type C particle, is known to be widespread in the cat population.

Although some authors [34, 75] have suggested that the cat represents a good animal model for use in the study of mammary cancer in women, the cat has not been utilized in the carcinogenic testing of contraceptive steroids. In this respect, HERNANDEZ et al. [36] reported that two of five privately owned cats that received medroxyprogesterone acetate as a contraceptive for $3\frac{1}{2}$ and 5 years, respectively, developed adenocarcinomas within 2—4 years after the last drug injection.

Dogs

Mammary tumors represent the most common form of neoplastic disease in the female dog. Despite their common occurrence, accurate data on the incidence of mammary neoplasms in the canine population are difficult to obtain. The only report on the incidence of mammary tumors in a general population of dogs was that of DORN et al. [18], who stated that the annual incidence of histologically malignant tumors was approximately 200 per 100,000 female dogs in the San Francisco Bay area of California. Numerous reports indicate that the relative frequency of mammary tumors as compared to other canine tumors is very high, ranging from 10% to 40% of all tumors (see review by HAMILTON [32]). An additional problem encountered in calculating the frequency of mammary tumors is the common occurrence of multiple mammary tumors in the same dog and even in the same gland. FOWLER et al. [28] reported that 44% of 154 dogs with mammary neoplasia had multiple tumors of different histogenetic types. MULLIGAN [57] reported that up to 10% of the dogs with mixed tumors had coexisting carcinomas in the same or separate mammary glands. CAMERON and FAUKLIN, [8], using the whole-mount technique in the study of mammary glands, reported that of 654 glandular nodules in six dogs, 14% were considered neoplasms, 15% were normal hyperplastic nodules, 8% were inflammatory nodules, and 56% were hyperplastic nodules with disproportionate epithelial proliferations. The dog has five pairs of mammary glands, and most studies have shown that 50%—60% of the tumors occur in the two most caudal glands [32]. MULLIGAN [55] suggested that the propensity for the development of neoplasms in the caudal glands was associated with an increased affinity for estrogen by these glands. The more recent studies of WARNER [73] and of CAMERON and FAULKIN [8] indicate that the two most caudal glands comprise 60% of the mammary tissue in the dog, which is probably the reason for the large number of neoplasms in these glands.

Susceptibility of different breeds to mammary neoplasia has been studied by numerous authors. Fox terriers, Boston terriers, and dachshunds [55] have been reported to have a greater incidence of the disease than expected. FRYE et al. in 1967 [29] also reported that the dachshund, on a statistical basis, had a larger number of tumors than other breeds. Conversely, the disease was reported to be less frequent in the collie [29], the boxer [39], and the chihuahua [18]. ANDERSEN's studies [2] in beagles suggested that this breed has an unusually high incidence of the disease, as 38% of the female beagles maintained in an experimental colony developed mammary tumors during the first 8 years of life and mammary cancer resulted in the death of 27% of the animals over a 13-year period. FRYE et al.'s [29] study, however, failed to demonstrate a statistically significant increase in mammary tumors in pet beagles as compared to other breeds. Recently DORN and SCHNEIDER [17] reported that inbreeding coefficients were higher in 11 breeds of dogs with mammary cancer, yet these coefficients were not statistically different from those of dogs with other types of cancers or dogs without tumors.

Mammary neoplasia of the dog is principally a disease of middle aged or old animals. Tumors are uncommon before 2–6 years of age but incidence increases rapidly after 6 years with a peak by the age of 10–11 [18]. Although benign tumors have been described as occurring at an earlier age [19] than malignant tumors, most studies involving large numbers of tumors have shown that this difference in age is not statistically significant [29, 54].

Mammary neoplasia of the dog is principally a disease of middle aged or old animals. Tumors carcinoma to pleomorphic neoplasms containing bone and cartilage interspersed among epithelial and myoepithelial cells. The neoplasms are frequently accompanied by a large amount of fibrous stroma and dilated or cystic ducts. These diverse histologic patterns, coupled with the tendency to develop multiple nodules with variable histologic features within the same dog or same gland, have resulted in a great deal of confusion as to the classification of neoplasms, hyperplasias, and dysplasias. The small number of prospective studies on dogs with mammary tumors has limited the knowledge available on the biologic behavior of the different histologic types of tumors. As would be expected, most of the literature on mammary lesions in dogs has concentrated on malignant tumors and limited emphasis has been placed on the characterization of benign tumors and hyperplastic lesions.

The variable histologic patterns seen in canine mammary tumors are largely attributed to the myoepithelial cells. These cells, located in the ducts and acini, have a marked propensity to proliferate in this species. In many tumors these cells produce large amounts of mucopolysaccharides and may undergo metaplasia to cartilage, which ultimately results in formation of osteoid and bone in some tumors. The presence of cartilage or bone in canine mammary neoplasms (mixed tumors) is extremely common and is seen in 25%–50% of the tumors (see review by HAMILTON [32]). It is now generally accepted that the origin of most mucoid and cartilaginous tissue in canine mammary tumors results from the metaplasia of the myeoepithelial cell (see review by PULLEY [63]).

Until recently, most authors have used a combination of histogenetic and histologic systems to classify canine mammary tumors [14, 24, 28, 53–55, 57]. The terminology varies considerably in the different classification systems and a standard classification has not been fully adopted. In 1958, COTCHIN [14] gave an elegant description of mammary tumors in 424 dogs, in which 187 tumors were malignant and 249 benign. Of the malignant tumors 88 were classified as carcinomas, 73 as sarcomas, and 27 as malignant complex tumors. The carcinomas were subdivided into squamous cell, duct carcinoma, adenocarcinoma, sclerosing carcinoma, solid carcinoma, and anaplastic carcinoma.

COTCHIN [14] proposed the use of the terms "simple" and "complex" to describe many of the benign mammary tumors in dogs. The term "simple" was applied to lesions composed of one cell type. Complex benign lesions were composed of true epithelial cells and an "interposed" cell (cells between the secretory epithelium and the basement membrane presumed to be myoepithelial cells). These complex lesions had a tendency to develop mucoid, cartilaginous, or bony areas. The largest series of canine neoplasms (1366) reported was classified by MOULTON et al. [54] as shown in Table 1. The 541 carcinomas reported were further subdivided into lobular (14%), papillary (15%), solid (18%), infiltrating (46%), and squamous (3%) types. Both MULLIGAN [55, 57] and FOWLER et al. [28] have preferred to emphasize a

Table 1. Classification of 1366 canine mammary tumors (adapted from MOULTON et al. [54])

Tumor type	Percentage
Adenomas	5.1
Myoepitheliomas	1.1
Benign mixed tumors	45.1
Malignant mixed tumors	8.5
Carcinomas (all types)	39.7
Fibrosarcomas	0.1
Sarcomas	0.5

histogenetic approach to the classification of carcinomas. They reported that the major portion of the malignant epithelial neoplasms were either ductal or lobular carcinomas. FOWLER et al. [28] considered sarcomas of the mammary gland to be forms of malignant myoepithelial tumors that could appear as osteosarcomas, fibrosarcomas, or combinations of the two.

The lack of a standardized classification for mammary tumors and that of other types of tumors of domestic animals has been recognized by investigators throughout the world. In response to this need, the World Health Organization (WHO) organized a number of expert committees and comparative oncology centers in several countries in 1966. One of the major purposes of this WHO program was to develop an international classification system for tumors of domestic animals. In late 1974, a classification system for ten organ systems was published that included mammary gland tumors and dysplasias. The classification for mammary tumors was prepared by HAMPE and MISDORP [33] from over 800 mammary lesions collected from centers located in several countries. The WHO classification system is based solely on the histology of the lesion. One of the principal differences from previous classifications of mammary gland tumors was the inclusion of the myoepithelial cell as a component of some types of carcinomas. Carcinomas containing a myoepithelial cell component were termed "complex," (Figs. 21 and 22), contrasted with "simple" carcinomas composed solely of luminal or secretory cells (Figs. 23 and 24). The WHO system also included a classification of hyperplastic and apparently benign tumors. MISDORP and HART [46] used the WHO classification in reporting the biologic behavior of 296 malignant tumors. BOSTOCK [5] also used the WHO classification in reporting behavior in a series of benign and malignant tumors in 320 dogs. The WHO system has also been used to classify lesions of the mammary gland in dogs treated with contraceptive steroids by the Central Repository for Tissue Evaluation of Contraceptive Steroids located at the Armed Forces Institute of Pathology, Washington, D. C. In conjunction with the contraceptive steroid studies, 939 spontaneous canine tumors and dysplasias in the Registry of Veterinary Pathology were classified by the WHO system. The Registry cases (Table 2), represent spontaneous lesions submitted for consultation from pathologists throughout the United States since 1944. Most reports indicate that about 50% of all canine mammary tumors are histologically malignant [14, 29, 54]. In some studies, over 70% of all tumors were classed as malignant [5, 69], but the exact percentage of histologically malignant neoplasms that metastasize has not been firmly established because of the lack of prospective follow-up studies. In 1975, BOSTOCK [5] reported that of 227 dogs with carcinomas, 43% died as a result of the disease within 2 years and the median survival time was 70 weeks. Survival was correlated with the degree of invasiveness of the tumors in both simple and complex carcinomas. Dogs with

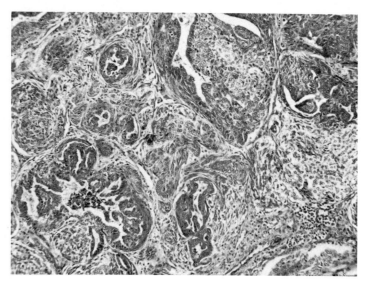

Fig. 21. Complex tubular adenocarcinoma, dog. AFIP Neg. No. 77-5276, H & E, × 100

anaplastic carcinomas had the shortest survival time and highest mortality rate, followed by those with solid, tubular, and papillary carcinomas. FOWLER et al. [28] reported the biologic behavior of 271 mammary gland tumors in 154 bitches: infiltrative ductal and lobular carcinomas exhibited the highest rate of metastasis in these studies. Survival times after initial diagnosis have also been reported by MISDORP and HART [46] for malignant tumors as classified by the WHO system. Over 75% of the 253 dogs with malignant tumors died within 2

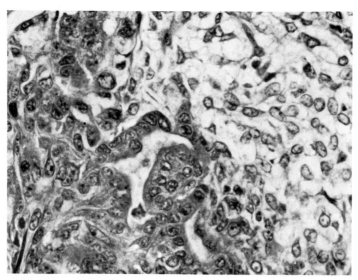

Fig. 22. Complex adenocarcinoma shown in Figure 21, illustrating solid areas of vacuolated myoepithelial cells and secretory glandular component. AFIP Neg. No. 77-5297, H & E, × 485

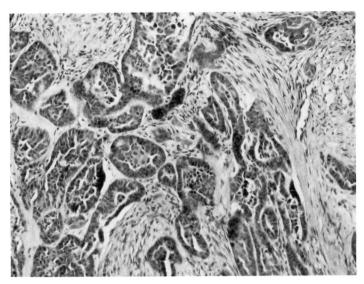

Fig. 23. Simple tubular carcinoma, dog. AFIP Neg. No. 77-5321, H & E, × 115

years of the initial tumor diagnosis. The histologic type was correlated with the degree of malignancy in the following descending order: sarcomas, simple carcinomas, complex carcinomas. Surprisingly, involvement of regional lymph nodes could not be correlated with the length of survival. In earlier studies by MISDORP et al. [47–49], dogs with simple adenocarcinomas had a median survival time of 14 months after diagnosis versus 20 months for complex adenocarcinomas. Dogs with solid carcinomas, both simple and complex, had

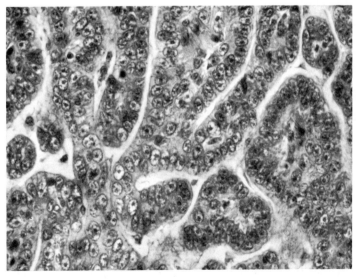

Fig. 24. Simple papillary adenocarcinoma, dog. AFIP Neg. No. 77-5293, H & E, × 485

Table 2. Histologic types of 939 spontaneous canine mammary tumors in the Registry of Veterinary Pathology, Armed Forces Institute of Pathology; classified by the WHO system

Histologic type	Number	Histologic type	Number
Benign or apparently benign dysplasias	51	**Carcinoma**	355
		Simple tubular adenocarcinoma	63
Cyst, nonpapillary	2	Simple papillary adenocarcinoma	38
Cyst, papillary	4	Simple papillary cystic adenocarcinoma	16
Duct ectasia	3	Simple solid carcinoma	43
Lobular hyperplasia	38	Simple (combined – tubular/papillary/	49
Intraductal hyperplasia	3	solid) carcinoma	
Fibrosclerosis	1	Complex tubular adenocarcinoma	71
		Complex papillary adenocarcinoma	5
Benign tumors	470	Complex solid carcinoma	16
		Complex (combined – tubular/papillary/	14
Adenoma	57	solid) carcinoma	
Papilloma	30	Squamous cell carcinoma	14
Papillomatosis	12	Spindle cell carcinoma	2
Complex adenoma	122	Anaplastic carcinoma	24
Benign mixed tumor	223		
Fibroadenoma	4	**Malignant mixed tumor**[a]	15
Benign soft tissue tumor	22		
		Carcinosarcoma	2
		Sarcoma	46
		Osteosarcoma	22
		Fibrosarcoma	11
		Undifferentiated	6
		Other	7

[a] Tumors containing both mesenchymal and epithelial components in which the epithelial component was interpreted as malignant. Some investigators could interpret these as carcinomas arising in benign mixed tumors.

median survival times of 9 and 12 months, respectively. Dogs with anaplastic carcinomas had the shortest median survival time (7 months) followed by dogs with sarcomas (10 months) and dogs with malignant mixed tumors termed carcinosarcomas (18 months).

It has been recognized for many years [16, 64] that the ovaries play an important role in the development of canine mammary tumors and that ovariectomized animals have a lower frequency of the disease. The effect of the ovary on the development of mammary tumors occurs early in the dog's life [7, 25, 56, 65], as ovariectomy markedly reduces the risk of tumor development if performed at an early age. SCHNEIDER et al. [65] showed in retrospective studies on 93 ovariectomized bitches and 87 matched controls that the reduced risk for the development of mammary tumors was directly dependent on the time of ovariectomy relative to the initial and subsequent estrous cycles the dog hat experienced. Ovariectomy before the first estrus reduced the risk of tumor development to 0.5%, after the first estrus, to 8%, and after the second estrus, to 26%. Ovariectomy after the dog reached 2½ years of age had no effect on the frequency of the disease.

The effect of the administration of exogenous estrogen, progesterone, and related contraceptive steroidal compounds is of immense interest because the dog serves as one of the test animals for carcinogenic testing of contraceptive steroid drugs in the United States. These long-term studies (up to 7 years) are conducted in accordance with FDA guidelines [4], generally at 1—2, 10, or 25 times the recommended human dosage. Results of some of these canine studies have shown that certain contraceptive steroids produce large numbers of mammary nodules. This finding has resulted in the removal of some compounds from the market and the curtailment of investigations of other compounds. Those drugs removed from the market include chlormadinone acetate, medroxyprogesterone acetate, and megestrol acetate [26]. Drugs that have been shown to produce mammary nodules in the dog include ethynerone, chloroethynyl norgestrel, and anagestone acetate [74]. Progesterone has also been shown to produce similar nodules in the dog [12, 70]. The development of nodules is dose related, and dogs receiving the highest dose levels (25 times the human dose) have the largest number of lesions. With dose levels 10 times greater, the number of nodules generally exceeds that observed in control animals, while at dose levels of 1—2 times greater, nodules are observed in numbers comparable to controls. In contrast, the nonhalogenated 19-nor-testosterone derivatives norgestrel, norethindrone, norethynodrel, and ethynodiol diacetate, have not produced mammary nodules in the canine mammary gland. Likewise, the estrogens given in combination with these 19-nortestosterone drugs have not produced nodules in the canine mammary gland.

The suitability of the dog as a test animal has been often questioned [9, 15, 37, 38, 60, 61, 70]. Critics point out that the canine estrous cycle — one cycle every 6—9 months with a long period of anestrus (3—6 months) — is remarkably different from that of women and that the frequency of administration of drugs to dogs as used in women (3 weeks on, 1 week off cycle) is inappropriate. Furthermore, some critics feel that the dog is unusually sensitive to progestins and that many of the nodules produced are not true tumors. These critics point out that many nodules undergo spontaneous regression. Some investigators have also questioned whether or not the finding of the benign mixed tumor of dogs frequently observed in these studies is significant, pointing out that this tumor is basically peculiar to the dog and is rarely observed in women. Despite the controversies surrounding the mammary nodules in treated dogs, reports describing the pathology of the nodules were extremely limited until recently. VALLANCE and CAPEL-EDWARDS [70] reported fibroadenomas in two dogs treated with progesterone and NELSON et al. [61] described the pathology of 38 nodules in dogs treated with megestrol acetate and 22 nodules in dogs treated with chlormadinone acetate in studies conducted from 2—4 years. In NELSON's studies [61] the nodules ranged in size from 1 mm to 7.5 cm in diameter. Although 60 nodules were present at necropsy, 159 nodules were observed by palpation studies during the course of the experiment, which included four transitory nodules in control dogs. Histologically, 39 of the 60 nodules were classified as hyperplasias. Nine nonproliferative lesions were described. Many of the smaller nodules (less than 1 cm) were regarded as non-neoplastic and were undergoing regressive changes. Nine benign mixed tumors containing bone or cartilage were observed in dogs receiving the highest dose levels. One animal developed an adenocarcinoma, which metastasized to the regional lymph nodes.

The lack of studies on the pathology of mammary gland nodules in dogs administered contraceptive steroids prompted the establishment of the Central Repository for Tissue Evaluation of Contraceptive Steroids at the Armed Forces Institute of Pathology in 1972 in a cooperative effort with the National Institute of Child Health and Human Development. Using studies from the Repository, GILES et al. [31] recently reported on the pathology of 934 mammary nodules from dogs treated with three drugs in combination with mestranol: anagestone, chloroethynyl norgestrel, and ethynerone (Table 3). Mammary lesions from control and mestranol-treated dogs were also studied. The vast majority of the lesions reported consisted of mammary hyperplasias and benign tumors. Of the 934 nodules, 31% were classified as lobular or intraductular hyperplasias, 21%, as simple adenomas, 25%, as complex adenomas, 5%, as benign mixed tumors, and 4%, as malignant in that they had definite invasive features or had metastasized (Table 4). The balance of the nodules were mammary dysplasias consisting of ductal ectasias, cysts, and fibrosclerotic nodules. Six percent of the nodules were from nonmammary tissue. Hyperplastic lesions (Fig. 25) both lobular and intraductal, were similar to the spontaneous mammary gland hyperplasias in the dog. The mean size of these hyperplastic lesions was 4.0 mm, with a range of 1–30 mm. The number of simple adenomas reported by GILES et al. [31] in the contraceptive-treated dogs formed a higher percrcentage of this type of tumor than is generally reported in spontaneous tumors. In addition, GILES et al. [31] reported that 82 (48%) of the simple adenomas were of the basaloid type. The pathology of the 82 basaloid adenomas was described in detail by KWAPIEN et al. [45]; the adenomas were considered drug related, as this type of tumor had not been described previously as a spontaneous tumor of the mammary gland of the dog. The neoplasm occurred only in progestin-treated dogs receiving the mid and higher dosages. The basaloid adenomas were generally small (with mean diameter of 6.7 mm). The tumor appeared to arise in both the lobules and ducts and was composed of relatively small, uniform

Table 3. Nodules in the mammary gland region of beagle dogs on long-term investigational contraceptive steroid drugs (modified from GILES et al. [31])

Drug	Dose mg/kg/day	No. dogs with nodules at necropsy/ No. dogs in group	No. nodules palpated during the study	No. nodules coalescing	No. of nodules at necropsy
Anagestone plus	0.44	13/13	198	13	149
mestranol[a]	1.10	12/13	161	4	135
Chlorethynyl	0.084	7/16	32	0	17
norgestrel	0.42	16/17	183	3	176
plus mestranol[b]	1.05	16/16	280	25	248
Ethynerone plus	0.084	2/16	15	0	4
mestranol[b]	0.42	5/16	25	0	9
	1.05	15/17	199	5	153
Ethynerone	1.00	9/18	50	0	26
Mestranol	0.02	0/15	1	0	0
	0.05	4/15	12	0	8
Control	–	6/18	40	0	9

[a] Ratio of progestin to mestranol was 10 : 1.
[b] Ratio of progestin to mestranol was 20 : 1.

Table 4. Classification of 934 nodules in the mammary gland region of dogs administered oral contraceptive steroids (modified from GILES et al. [31])

Drug	Dose mg/kg/day	Non-mammary nodules	Benign mammary dysplasias	Hyperplasias (lobular and intraductal)	Simple adenomas	Complex adenomas	Benign mixed tumors	Malignant tumors No. of nodules/No. of dogs
Anagestone plus mestranol[a]	0.44	3	11	54	17	34	19	11/3
	1.10	8	3	58	28	27	9	2/1
Chloroethynyl norgestrel[b]	0.084	3	5	6	3	—	—	—
	0.42	3	8	55	56	46	8	—
plus mestranol[b]	1.05	6	4	65	42	113	12	6/4
Ethynerone plus mestranol[b]	0.084	2	—	2	—	—	—	—
	0.42	6	1	2	—	—	—	—
	1.05	22	28	39	36	14	—	14/1
Ethynerone	1.00	3	5	7	9	1	1	—
Mestranol	0.02	—	—	—	—	—	—	—
	0.05	4	—	3	1	—	—	—
Control	—	2	—	5	—	—	2	—
Percent of all nodules		6.5	7.0	31.4	20.8	25.4	5.3	3.6

[a] Ratio of progestin to mestranol was 10 : 1.
[b] Ratio of progestin to mestranol was 20 : 1.

cells surrounded by very delicate stroma (Fig. 26). Squamous differentiation with keratin formation was also a common microscopic feature of the tumor. The most common neoplasm in the large series described by GILES et al. [31] was the complex adenoma. These tumors varied markedly in size, ranging from 2 mm to 28 cm, with a mean diameter of just under 2 cm. The complex adenomas were composed of an admixture of secretory and myeoepithe-

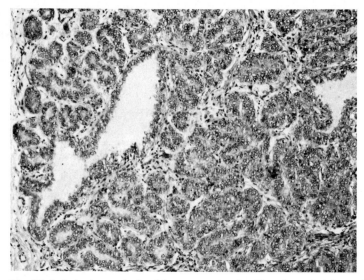

Fig. 25. Lobular hyperplasia of the mammary gland in a dog administered 0.084 mg ethynerone plus mestranol/kg body wt. AFIP Neg. No. 77-5506, H & E, × 40

lial cells in varying proportions (Fig. 27). They were frequently multinodular in nature with some having prominent areas of fibrosis and central necrosis. GILES et al. [31] felt that many of the complex adenomas had formed by coalescence of adjacent smaller nodules. Fifty-one benign mixed tumors were reported in this series. These tumors, by definition, had areas of cartilage and/or bone formation (Fig. 28). In noncartilaginous or nonosseous areas, their morphology was essentially identical to that of many of the complex adenomas. The mean

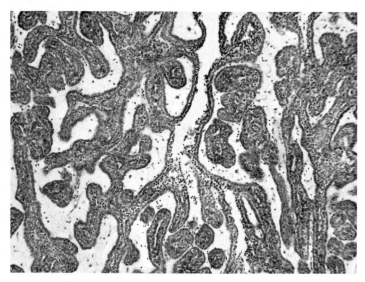

Fig. 26. Basaloid adenoma in a dog administered 1.1 mg anagestone acetate/kg body wt. AFIP Neg. No. 76-223, H & E, × 130

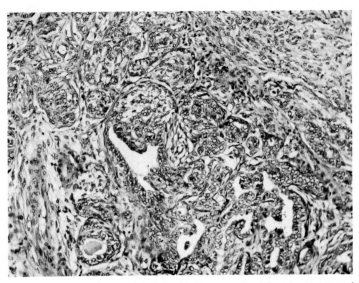

Fig. 27. Complex adenoma composed of secretory epithelial cells forming glandular structures and spindle-shaped myoepithelial cells, dog administered 1.05 mg ethynerone plus mestranol/kg body wt. AFIP Neg. No. 74-10564, H & E, × 130

size of the mixed tumors was only slightly larger than the complex adenomas, 2.1 cm versus 1.9 cm. Thirty-three malignant mammary nodules were described in nine dogs. All dogs with malignant tumors had received progestin/mestranol combinations; four dogs in each group received mid and high doses of anagestone and chloroethynyl norgestrel. One high-dose

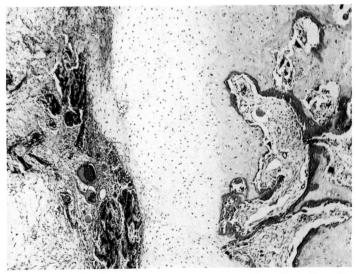

Fig. 28. Benign mixed mammary tumor illustrating large areas of cartilage and bone formation, dog administered 1.05 mg chloroethynyl norgestrel plus mestranol/kg body wt. AFIP Neg. No. 77-2893, H & E, × 65

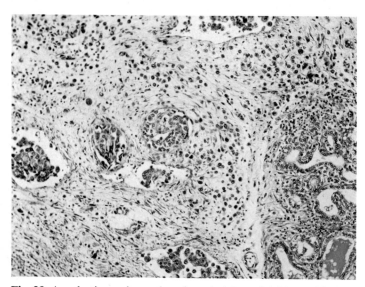

Fig. 29. Anaplastic carcinoma in a dog administered 1.05 mg chloroethynyl norgestrel plus mestranol/kg body wt. Large anaplastic cells have diffusely infiltrated edematous stroma and are present in dilated lymphatics. AFIP Neg. No. 76-10070, H & E, × 100

animal to which ethynerone was administered developed 20 malignant sarcomatous nodules. Carcinomas included solid types, tubular adenocarcinomas, squamous cell, and anaplastic carcinomas. Anaplastic carcinomas (Figs. 29 and 30) were present in five of the nine dogs with malignant neoplasms.

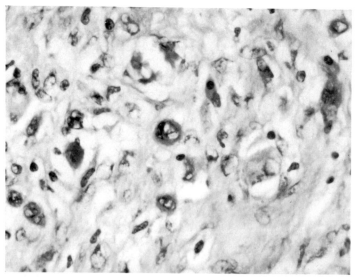

Fig. 30. Large individualized cells of an anaplastic carcinoma of the mammary gland. From a dog administered 1.05 mg chloroethynyl norgestrel plus mestranol/kg body wt. AFIP Neg. No. 77-5504, H & E, × 485

Nonhuman Primates

Mammary tumors in the nonhuman primate have been uncommon; only 12 have been reported in the literature (see review by APPLEBY [3]). However, only a very limited number of nonhuman primates have been observed clinically throughout their normal life span. Interest in neoplasia of the mammary gland remains high, for the rhesus monkey now serves as a test animal for the carcinogenic testing of contraceptive steroids in the United States. Mammary tumors have been described in five rhesus monkeys (*Macaca mulatta*), two bush babies (*Galago crassicaudatus*), a single green monkey (*Ceropithecus sabacus*), one baboon (*Papio homadryas*), one orangutan (*Pongo pygmacus*), one mandrill (*Mandrillis sphinx*), and one tree shrew (*Tapaia glis*). Where known, the age of the animals ranged from 5 to 15 years. Four rhesus monkeys with malignant tumors were between 8 and 10 years of age.

Eight of the 12 tumors reported were classified as carcinomas, which included four adenocarcinomas, one ductal carcinoma, one squamous cell carcinoma, and two carcinomas of unspecified type. The two tumors in the Galagos that metastasized included a spindle cell carcinoma, probably of myoepithelial cell origin, and a malignant mixed tumor. Metastases were also reported in four of the five carcinomas occurring in the rhesus monkey; an RNA virus was subsequently isolated from one of these [11]. One adenocarcinoma occurred in a rhesus monkey following irradiation. Of particular interest was a widely metastasizing ductal carcinoma that developed in one of six monkeys that were under study with the contraceptive steroid Enovid-E, norethynodrel and mestranol, which had been administered for 18 months at the recommended human dosage [44]. In addition to the previously described malignant mammary tumors in nonhuman primates, the histologic features of a single mammary lesion termed nodular hyperplasia was described in a rhesus monkey that served as a control in a study of contraceptive steroids [59].

Mammary gland lesions, other than the single carcinoma reported by KIRSCHSTEIN et al. [44] in nonhuman primates administered contraceptive steroids, have been limited to intraductal

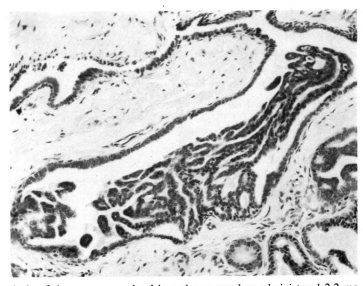

Fig. 31. Intraductal hyperplasia of the mammary gland in a rhesus monkey administered 2.2 mg anagestone acetate plus mestranol/kg body wt. AFIP Neg. No. 77-2885, H & E, × 180

hyperplasias reported by GEIL and LAMAR in 1976 [30] in biopsies from rhesus monkeys administered ethynerone, chloroethynyl norgestrel, anagestone, and/or mestranol (Fig. 31). The intraductal lesion was not seen in biopsies from four monkeys serving as controls in these studies. A similar intraductal lesion was observed in a specimen from the breast of a control monkey studied at the AFIP Central Tissue Repository for the Evaluation of Contraceptive Steroids. This center has also observed the same lesion in rhesus monkeys treated with medroxyprogesterone acetate.

In comparison with the dog, the induction of persistent mammary gland nodules in monkeys administered contraceptive steroids is remarkably different. DRILL et al. [20] reported that 96 monkeys receiving either norethynodrel or ethynodiol diacetate for 5 years at 1, 10, and 50 times the recommended human dosage failed to develop palpable mammary lesions. GEIL and LAMAR [30] reported that transitory small mammary nodules occurred in 23 monkeys treated with either ethynerone/mestranol, chloroethynyl norgestrel/mestranol, ethynerone, or anagestone. The size of the nodules was generally 1—2 mm in diameter, with the largest nodule reported as a flattened 6-mm mass that subsequently underwent complete regression. These investigators also noted that one control monkey and two monkeys receiving mestranol had palpable mammary nodules during 8 years of treatment and observation. The histologic appearance of these palpable mammary nodules was not correlated with the intraductal hyperplasia seen in random mammary gland biopsies from the same groups of monkeys discussed in the preceding paragraph.

Summary

The study of mammary neoplasms in animals and the use of experimental procedures to influence their development and progression has provided a great deal of insight into mammary carcinogenesis. Although the mouse, rat, cat, and dog develop mammary tumors with a sufficiently high frequency for use in experimental studies, none of these animals provide an ideal model for the study of the disease in women. Each species, including man, show certain unique aspects of the disease; yet, all share common features. Murine mammary tumors are primarily virus induced and provide an excellent laboratory animal model for studying genetic, immunologic, and hormonal interactions of virus-induced mammary tumors, a mechanism that could be operative in other species, including women. The development of mammary tumors in rats has been shown to be markedly altered by known chemical carcinogens. This property has favored the extensive use of this species in the testing of a variety of chemicals for carcinogenic properties. Mammary neoplasms in the cat perhaps most closely resemble the disease in women, but this model system has not been adequately exploited for this purpose. To effectively study the disease in cats would require long-term studies, since the mammary tumors occur in relatively old cats. The canine mammary neoplasm also occurs in older animals. Its use in comparative studies has been limited primarily to the carcinogenic testing of contraceptive steroids when it was recognized that this species develops a significant number of proliferative mammary lesions after 2—4 years of drug administration. Subsequent studies have clearly demonstrated that high doses of 17 α-hydroxyprogesterone derivatives and halogenated 19-nortestosterone derivatives produce a wide variety of proliferative lesions in the canine mammary gland which range from hyperplasias to metastasizing neoplasms. Nonhalogenated derviatives of 19-nortestosterones (presently marketed compounds) have not been shown to produce excessive mammary nodules in the dog even when administered at the higher doses; however, reports in the literature describing the ongoing findings of long-term studies with these drugs are limited. Minimal chemical alteration of the 19-nortestosterone derivatives such s halogenation at the 17th position is sufficient to make these compounds carcinogenic in the dog. Estrogens when administered alone do not produce excessive neoplasms in the dog. This is in contrast to the effects of estrogen in rodents, which at high doses, either alone or in combination with progestins, may promote the development of mammary tumors. Studies on the effects of contraceptive steroids on the mammary gland of nonhuman primates are incomplete. The significance of the intraductal hyperplasia observed microscopically in biopsies from nonhuman primates treated with 17 α-hydroxyprogesterone derivatives and halogenated 19-testosterone derivatives is unknown, but it is of sufficient interest to warrant the continued observation of these animals for several years.

It is inappropriate to extrapolate the findings in experimental animals directly to man, but in the absence of data on humans, animal studies must be used when it is necessary to make predictive judgments on factors that could influence the occurrence of a disease in man. In the case of contraceptive steroids, early animal studies indicated that some drugs could have carcinogenic properties. Since these drugs have now been administered to women for a number of years, future epidemiologic studies should permit the evaluation of their carcinogenic potential without reliance on animal data.

References

1. Allen, H. L.: Feline mammary hypertrophy. Vet. Pathol. *10*, 501—508 (1973)
2. Andersen, A. C.: Parameters of mammary gland tumors in aging beagles (abstract). JAVMA *147*, 1653 (1965)
3. Appleby, E. C., Keymer, I. F., Hime, J. M.: Three cases of suspected mammary neoplasia in nonhuman primates. J. Comp. Pathol. *84*, 351—364 (1974)
4. Berliner, V. R.: U.S. Food and Drug Administration requirements for toxicity testing of contraceptive products. In: Pharmacological Models in Contraceptive Development, WHO Symposium, Geneva: Bureau FDA, 1973, pp. 240—253
5. Bostock, D. E.: The prognosis following the surgical excision of canine mammary neoplasms. Eur. J. Cancer *11*, 386—396 (1975)
6. Bradley, C. J., Kledzik, G. S., Meites, J.: Prolactin and estrogen dependency of rat mammary cancers at early and late stages of development. Cancer Res. *36*, 319—324 (1976)
7. Brodey, R. S., Fidler, I. J., Howson, A. E.: The relationship of estrous irregularity, pseudopregnancy, and pregnancy to the development of canine mammary neoplasms. JAVMA *149*, 1047—1049 (1966)
8. Cameron, A. M., Faulkin, L. J., Jr.: Hyperplastic and inflammatory nodules in the canine mammary gland. J. Natl. Cancer Inst. *47*, 1277—1287 (1971)
9. Capel-Edwards, K., Hall, D. E., Fellowes, K. P., Vallance, D. K., Daview, M. J., Lamb, D., Robertson, W. B.: Long-term administration of progesterone to the female beagle dog. Toxicol. Appl. Pharmacol. *24*, 474—488 (1973)
10. Carcinogenicity Tests of Oral Contraceptives. A report by the Committee on Safety of Medicines. London: Her Majesty's Stationery Office, 1972
11. Chopra, H. C., Mason, M. M.: A new virus in a spontaneous mammary tumor of a rhesus monkey. Cancer Res. *30*, 2081—2086 (1970)
12. Coleman, M. E., Murchison, T. E., Frank, D.: Mammary nodules in dogs receiving Depo-Provera and progesterones: An interim progress report. Toxicol. Appl. Pharmacol. *37*, 181 (1976)
13. Cotchin, E.: Neoplasia in the cat. Vet. Rec. *69*, 425—434 (1957)
14. Cotchin, E.: Mammary neoplasms of the bitch. J. Comp. Pathol. *68*, 1—21 (1958)

15. Daniel, G. R.: Chlormadinone contraceptive withdrawn. Br. Med. J. *1*, 303 (1970)
16. De Vitta, J.: Mammary adenofibroma of the female dog. N. Am. Vet. *20*, 53—55 (1939)
17. Dorn, C. R., Schneider, R.: Inbreeding and canine mammary cancer: A retrospective study. J. Natl. Cancer Inst. *57*, 545—548 (1976)
18. Dorn, C. R., Taylor, D. O. N., Schneider, R., Hibbard, H. H., Klauber, M. R.: Survey of animal neoplasms in Alameda and Contra Costa counties, California. I. Cancer morbidity in dogs and cats from Alameda county. J. Natl. Cancer Inst. *40*, 307—318 (1968)
19. Drill, V. A.: Experimental and clinical studies on relationship of estrogens and oral contraceptives to breast cancer. In: Experimental Model Systems in Toxicology and Their Significance in Man, Proceedings of the European Society for the Study of Drug Toxicity. Zurich: 1973, Vol. XV, pp. 200—214
20. Drill, V. A., Martin, D. P., Hart, E. R., McConnell, R. G.: Effect of oral contraceptives on the mammary glands of rhesus monkeys: A preliminary report. J. Natl. Cancer Inst. *52*, 1655—1657 (1974)
21. Dunn, T. B.: Morphology of mammary tumors in mice. In: The Physiopathology of Cancer. Hamburger, F. (Ed.). New York: Harper (Hoeber), 1959, pp. 38—84
22. Durbin, P. W., Williams, M. H., Jeung, N., Arnold, J. S.: Development of spontaneous mammary tumors over the life-span of female Charles River (Sprague-Dawley) rats. The influence of ovariectomy, thyroidectomy and adrenalectomy-ovariectomy. Cancer Res. *26*, 400—426 (1966)
23. Feldman, D. G., Gross, L.: Electron microscopic study of spontaneous mammary carcinomas in cats and dogs: Virus-like particles in cat mammary carcinomas. Cancer Res. *31*, 1261—1267 (1971)
24. Fidler, J., Brodey, R. S.: A necropsy study of canine malignant mammary neoplasms. JAVMA *151*, 710—715 (1967)
25. Fidler, I. J., Abt, D. A., Brodey, R. S.: The biological behavior of canine mammary neoplasms. JAVMA *151*, 1311—1318 (1967)
26. Finkel, M. J., Berliner, V. R.: The extrapolation of experimental findings (animal to man): The dilemma of the systemically administered contraceptives. Presented at 62nd Annual Meeting of the IAP, Washington, D. C., pp. 13—18 (1973)
27. Foulds, L.: The histologic analysis of mammary tumors of mice. II. The histology of responsiveness and progression. The origins of tumors. J. Natl. Cancer Inst. *17*, 713—752 (1956)
28. Fowler, E. H., Wilson, G. P., Koestner, A.: Biologic behavior of canine mammary neoplasms based on a histogenetic classification. Vet. Pathol. *77*, 212—229 (1974)
29. Frye, F. L., Dorn, C. R., Taylor, D. O. N., Hibbard, H. H., Klauber, M. R.: Characteristics of canine mammary gland tumor cases. Anim. Hospital *3*, 1—12 (1967)
30. Geil, R. G., Lamar, J. K.: FDA studies of estrogen, progestogen and estrogen/progestogen. Inter. Res. & Develop. Corp., Mattawan, Michigan and the FDA, Rockville, Maryland. Presented at the Third Annual NCTR Res. Symp., Little Rock, Arkansas (1976)
31. Giles, R. C., Kwapien, R., Geil, R. G., Casey, H. W.: Mammary nodules in beagle dogs administered investigational oral contraceptive steroids. J. Natl. Cancer Inst. *60*, 1351—1364 (1978)
32. Hamilton, J. M.: Comparative aspects of mammary tumors. Adv. Cancer Res. *19*, 1—37 (1974)
33. Hampe, J. F., Misdorp, W.: International histological classification of tumours of domestic animals. IX. Tumours and dysplasias of the mammary gland. Bull. WHO *50*, 111—133 (1974)
34. Hayden, D. W., Nielsen, S. W.: Feline mammary tumours. J. Small Anim. Pract. *12*, 687—697 (1971)
35. Hayes, A.: Feline mammary gland tumors. Vet. Clin. N. Am. *7*, 205—212 (1977)
36. Hernandez, F. J., Fernandez, B. B., Chertack, M., Gage, P. A.: Feline Pract., pp. 45—48 (1975)

37. Hill, R.: Pre-clinical toxicity of steroid hormones: Recent experiences with estrogens and proges-
    togens in the dog. Adv. Steroid Biochem. Pharmacol. *3*, 29—38 (1972)
38. Hill, R., Dumas, K.: The use of dogs for studies of toxicity of contraceptive hormones. Acta
    Endocrinol. [Suppl] (Kbh) *185*, 74—84 (1974)
39. Howard, E. B., Nielsen, S. W.: Neoplasms of the boxer dog. Am. J. Vet. Res. *26*, 114, 1121—1131
    (1965)
40. Huggins, C., Briziarelli, G., Sutton, H.: Rapid induction of mammary carcinoma in the rat and the
    influence of hormones on the tumors. J. Exp. Med. *109*, 25—42 (1958)
41. Huggins, C., Grand, L. C., Brillantes, F. P.: Mammary cancer induced by a single feeding of
    polynuclear hydrocarbons and its suppression. Nature (London) *189*, 204—207 (1961)
42. Ihle, J. N., Arthur, L. O., Fine, D. L.: Autogenous immunity to mouse mammary tumor virus in
    mouse strains of high and low mammary tumor incidence. Cancer Res. *36*, 2840—2844
    (1976)
43. International Agency for Research on Cancer: IARC Monographs on the Evaluation of Carci-
    nogenic Risk of Chemicals to Man. Lyon, France, WHO Vol. VI, "Sex Hormones", 1974
44. Kirschstein, R. L., Rabbon, A. S., Rusten, G. W.: Infiltrating duct carcinoma of the mammary
    gland of a rhesus monkey after administration of an oral contraceptive: A preliminary report. J.
    Natl. Cancer Inst. *48*, 551—556 (1972)
45. Kwapien, R. P., Giles, R. C., Geil, R. G., Casey, H. W.: Basaloid adenomas of the mammary gland
    in beagle dogs administered investigation contraceptive steroids. J. Natl. Cancer Inst. *59*,
    933—939 (1977)
46. Misdorp, W., Hart, A. A. M.: Prognostic factors in canine mammary cancer. J. Natl. Cancer Inst.
    56, 779—786 (1976)
47. Misdorp, W., Cotchin, E., Hampe, J. F., Jabara, A. G., von Sandersleben, J.: Canine malignant
    mammary tumours. I. Sarcomas. Vet. Pathol. *8*, 99—117 (1971)
48. Misdorp, W., Cotchin, E., Hampe, J. F., Jabara, A. G., von Sandersleben, J.: Canine malignant
    mammary tumours. II. Adenocarcinomas, solid carcinomas and spindle cell carcinomas. Vet.
    Pathol. *9*, 447—470 (1972)
49. Misdorp, W., Cotchin, E., Hampe, J. F., Jabara, A. G., von Sandersleben, J.: Canine malignant
    mammary tumors. III. Special types of carcinomas, malignant mixed tumors. Vet. Pathol. *10*,
    241—256 (1973)
50. Moore, D. H., Charney, J., Holben, J. A.: Titrations of various mouse mammary tumor viruses in
    different mouse strains. J. Natl. Cancer Inst. *52*, 1757—1761 (1974)
51. Moore, D. H., Charney, J., Pullinger, B. D.: Mouse mammary tumor virus infectivity as a function
    of age at inoculation, breeding, and total lapsed time. J. Natl. Cancer Inst. *45*, 561—565
    (1970)
52. Moore, D. H., Holben, J. A., Charney, J.: Biologic characteristics of some mouse mammary tumor
    viruses. J. Natl. Cancer Inst. *57*, 889—896 (1976)
53. Moulton, J. E.: Tumors in Domestic Animals. Berkeley: Univ. Calif. Press, 1961, pp.
    179—189
54. Moulton, J. E., Taylor, D. O. N., Dorn, C. R., Andersen, A. C.: Canine mammary tumors. Pathol.
    Vet. *7*, 289—320 (1970)
55. Mulligan, R. M.: Neoplasms of the Dog. Baltimore: The Williams & Wilkins Company,
    1949
56. Mulligan, R. M.: Comparative pathology of human and canine cancer. Ann. N.Y. Acad. Sci. *108*,
    642—690 (1963)
57. Mulligan, R. M.: Mammary cancer in the dog: A study of 120 cases. Am. J. Vet. Res. *36*,
    1391—1396 (1975)
58. Nandi, S., McGrath, C. M.: Mammary neoplasia in mice. Adv. Cancer Res. *17*, 353—414
    (1973)
59. Nelson, L. W., Shott, L. D.: Mammary nodular hyperplasia in intact rhesus monkeys. Vet. Pathol.
    10, 130—134 (1973)

60. Nelson, L. W., Carlton, W. W., Weikel, J. H., Jr.: Canine mammary neoplasms and progestogens. JAMA *219*, 1601—1606 (1972)

61. Nelson, L. W., Weikel, J. H., Jr., Reno, F. E.: Mammary nodules in dogs during four years treatment with megestrol acetate or chlormadinone acetate. J. Natl. Cancer Inst. *51*, 1303—1311 (1973)

62. Nielsen, S. W.: The malignancy of mammary tumors in cats. N. Am. Vet. *April*, 245—252 (1952)

63. Pulley, L.: Ultrastructural and histochemical demonstration of myoepithelium in mixed tumors of the canine mammary gland. Am. J. Vet. Res. *34*, 1513—1522 (1973)

64. Riser, W. H.: Surgical removal of the mammary gland of the bitch. JAVMA *110*, 86—90 (1947)

65. Schneider, R., Dorn, C. R., Taylor, D. O. N.: Factors influencing canine mammary cancer development and postsurgical survival. J. Natl. Cancer Inst. *43*, 1249—1261 (1969)

66. Segaloff, A.: The role of the ovary in estrogen production of mammary cancer in the rat. Cancer Res. *34*, 2708—2710 (1974)

67. Sher, S. P.: Mammary tumors in control rats: Literature tabulation. Toxicol. Appl. Pharmacol. *22*, 562—588 (1972)

68. Stewart, H. L.: Comparative aspects of certain cancers. In: Cancer. Becker, F. F. (Ed.). New York: Plenum Publishing Corporation, 1976, Vol. IV, pp. 303—374

69. Uberreiter, O.: Neubildungen bei Tieren. Wien. Tieraerztl. Mschr. *47*, 805—832 (1960)

70. Vallance, D. K., Capel-Edwards, K.: Chlormadinone and mammary nodules. Br. Med. J. *2*, 221—222 (1971)

71. van Ebbenhorst Tengbergen, W. J. P. R.: Morphological classification of mammary tumours in the mouse. Pathol. Eur. *5*, 260—272 (1970)

72. van Nie, R., Dux, A.: Biological and morphological characteristics of mammary tumors in gr mice. J. Natl. Cancer Inst. *46*, 885—897 (1971)

73. Warner, M. R.: Age incidence and site distribution of mammary dysplasias in young beagle bitches. J. Natl. Cancer Inst. *57*, 57—61 (1976)

74. Wazeter, F. X., Geil, R. G., Berliner, V. R., Lamar, J. K.: Studies of tumorigenic and diabetogenic potential of certain oral contraceptive steroids in female dogs and monkeys. Toxicol. Appl. Pharmacol. *25*, 498 (1973)

75. Weijer, K., Head, K. W., Misdorp, W., Hampe, J. F.: Feline malignant mammary tumors. I. Morphology and biology: Some comparisons with human and canine mammary carcinomas. J. Natl. Cancer Inst. *49*, 1697—1704 (1972)

76. Welsch, C. W.: Interaction of estrogen and prolactin in spontaneous mammary tumorigenesis of the mouse. J. Toxicol. Environ. Health [Suppl.] *1*, 161—175 (1976)

77. Young, S., Hallowes, R. C.: Tumours of the mammary gland. In: Pathology of Tumours in Laboratory Animals. Vol. I. Tumours of the Rat. Turusov, V. S. (Ed.). Int. Agency for Res. on Cancer, Lyons, France: IARC Scientific Publication, No. 5, 1973, pp. 31—55

78. Young, S., Cowan, D. M., Sutherland, L. E.: The histology of induced mammary tumours in rats. J. Pathol. Bacteriol. *85*, 331—340 (1963)

Abnormalities of the Genital Tract Following Stilbestrol Exposure in Utero

Robert J. Kurman

Introduction

Seven years ago HERBST et al. [23] described eight cases of young women with clear-cell carcinoma of the vagina who had been exposed to diethylstilbestrol (DES) in utero. A Registry of Clear-Cell Adenocarcinoma of the Genital Tract in Young Females was subsequently established to centralize all available data on patients born after 1940, whether or not a history of DES exposure could be obtained, thereby facilitating rapid dissemination of information on the biologic behavior of the tumor and on appropriate therapeutic modalities. Presently, the Registry serves as a repository for clinical and pathologic data on over 300 women with this neoplasm. Reports from the Registry [20, 21] and additional publications from other sources [1, 7, 14, 24, 26, 32, 33, 39, 43, 48] have not only substantiated the association of vaginal and cervical clear-cell adenocarcinoma with intrauterine DES exposure, but have also shed light on a group of benign developmental anomalies resulting in a marked alteration of the lower genital tract. These include cervical or vaginal ridges and ectopic benign glandular epithelium in the vagina (adenosis) and cervix (ectropion) [19, 37, 40, 45]. These findings have widespread implications since it has been estimated that between 10,000 and 16,000 liveborn females per year between 1960 and 1970 were exposed to DES in utero in the United States [18]. DES was used as treatment for threatened and repeated abortions from 1945 into the early 1970s, not only in the United States but throughout other countries in Europe, South America, Africa, and Australia. Although it is still too early to be certain what the risk of developing carcinoma is, it appears at the present time that probably less than one exposed woman out of a thousand will develop carcinoma in adolescence [49], whereas almost all of the at risk population will develop one or more of the benign alterations [19, 21]. Since the mean latent period between exposure and development of carcinoma is 18 years, it is obvious that these women will have to be carefully followed for many years.

Embryology

In view of the apparent teratologic effect of DES on the cervix and vagina, it is pertinent to briefly review the embryology of the female genital tract [4, 9, 11, 12, 50]. The development of the human female reproductive tract begins at $\sim$ 6 weeks of gestation with the formation of the müllerian ducts which arise as invaginations of the coelomic epithelium near the genital ridges, the anlage of the primitive gonads. The müllerian ducts extend caudally toward the urogenital sinus in close proximity to the mesonephric (wolffian) ducts, crossing medial to the latter on entering the pelvis. The lower fused portion of the müllerian ducts penetrates the urogenital sinus at a point known as the müllerian tubercle. A focus of rapidly proliferating cells, interpreted as being of either mesonephric duct or urogenital sinus derivation, originates here and forms a solid core of tissue that obliterates the tubercle and extends cephalad, replacing the epithelium of the fused müllerian ducts. This solid core of tissue, called the vaginal plate, subsequently canalizes; the entire process is completed by the 5th month of gestation. In contrast to the human where the precise origin of the vaginal epithelial anlage remains uncertain, i.e., either mesonephric or urogenital sinus, the origin of the vagina in various laboratory animals has been established. Thus in the rat, mouse, and hamster it is derived to a varying degree from the müllerian and urogenital sinus epithelium with no contribution from the mesonephric ducts. Furthermore, whereas human vaginal development is complete by the 5th month of gestation, the vagina of the mouse continues to develop in the early neonatal period. It is evident that these differences must be appreciated when evaluating animal studies and attempting to extrapolate the findings to humans.

Investigations in Animals

Experimental evidence supports the theory that DES inhibits the replacement of the müllerian epithelium, thereby resulting in the aberrant location of glandular epithelium in the vagina and cervix. Thus GREENE, BURRIL and IVY [13] demonstrated an inhibition of the urogenital sinus, a proposed precursor of the vaginal plate, in the female offspring of rats that received DES during gestation. FORSBERG arrested the development of the caudal vagina of the rat and produced an increased number of mitoses in the müllerian epithelium of the vagina by administering estradiol to the mother during pregnancy [8]. He also induced glandlike downgrowths into the stroma of neonatal mice by the administration of estradiol-17β and DES [10].

Earlier work indicating that in utero exposure to DES was potentially carcinogenic was published by DUNN and GREEN who induced squamous cell carcinoma of the cervix of newborn female mice with injections of DES and produced epididymal cysts in the male offspring [5]. Similar results in male mice given DES have been reported by McLACHLAN et al. [30] who also found that 60% of these mice were sterile.

Clear-Cell Adenocarcinoma in Women

The patients range in age from 7 to 29 years with a mean of 18. Most often they present with vaginal bleeding or discharge although approximately 15% are asymptomatic. Almost three-fourths of the patients with vaginal neoplasms have tumors confined to the vaginal wall (stage I) whereas only 37% of the women with cervical tumors are stage I [20, 22]. Cytologic smears have been useful in the diagnosis of this tumor, but positive or suspicious smears have been reported in only 76% of patients [22, 47] (Table 1).

Approximately two-thirds of the patients in the Registry files have a history of maternal treatment with a nonsteroidal estrogen that includes DES, dienestrol, or hexestrol. An additional 10% received an unspecified medication for bleeding in pregnancy or previous miscarriage and approximately one-quarter have a negative history [20, 22] (Table 2). A progestational agent was used in conjunction with DES in 7% of the patients with tumors, indicating that the use of such drugs does not appear to mitigate the effect of DES [22]. It

Table 1. Cytologic findings in patients with vaginal and cervical clear-cell carcinoma[a]

Cytology	No.	%
Positive (IV or V)	49	76
Doubtful (II or III)	16	
Negative (I or II)	18	21
Unsatisfactory	2	
Total	85	

[a] A. L. HERBST et al.: Clear-cell adenocarcinoma of the vagina and cervix in girls: Analysis of 170 registry cases. Am. J. Obstet. Gynecol. *119*, 713–724 (1974).

should also be emphasized that there has not been a single example of a clear-cell carcinoma associated with a naturally occurring estrogen.

The dosages and duration of DES therapy have varied widely from as little as 1.5 mg to as much as 225 mg daily. The shortest duration of exposure has been 12 days. In all instances, however, treatment was initiated during the first half of pregnancy. At the present time, a clear-cut relationship has not been established between the dosage of DES or the duration of the exposure with the development of carcinoma [20, 22].

The vaginal and cervical tumors are similar in gross appearance; most are polypoid, nodular, or papillary, but some are flat or ulcerated (Fig. 1). The tumors display solid, papillary, tubular, and cystic patterns microscopically and are comprised of clear-cells containing abundant glycogen, hobnail cells characterized by a large nucleus with scant cytoplasm protruding into a lumen, and flattened cells (Figs. 2 and 3). When the tumor consists predominantly of cysts lined by flattened epithelium it may have a deceptively innocuous appearance. The identical tumor can occur in the endometrium [29, 44] and ovary [27, 34, 41], but in these sites there has never been an association with DES exposure and the neoplasms occur in older, generally postmenopausal women. Clear-cell carcinomas of the

Table 2. Maternal medication in pregnancy (144 patients)[a]

Pregnancy Rx.	Vagina	Cervix	Total	%
DES, Dienestrol, Hexestrol	56	28	84	65
DES, Dienestrol, Hexestrol c̄ Progestational agent	10	1	11	
Uns. med. for bleeding	11	8	19	
Total	77	37	114	78
No history of med.	12	18	30	22

[a] A. L. HERBST et al.: Clear-cell adenocarcinoma of the vagina and cervix in girls: Analysis of 170 registry cases. Am. J. Obstet. Gynecol. *119*, 713–724 (1974).

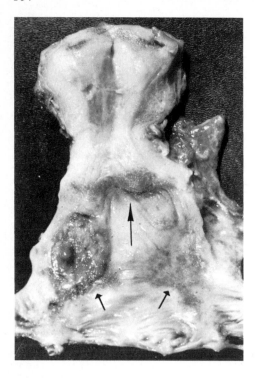

Fig. 1. Polypoid carcinoma on anterior wall of vagina. Adenosis borders the tumor and is present on the posterior wall (*small arrows*). There is an extensive cervical ectropion (*large arrow*). A. L. HERBST, and R. E. SCULLY: Cancer *25*, 745 (1970)

cervix have been reported with some frequency in women under 30 years of age prior to the DES era [15, 16].

In contrast there have been no more than 4 or 5 reports of this neoplasm in women in this age group in the vagina in the entire literature and therein lies one of the possible explanations why

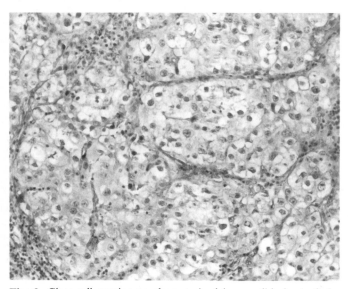

Fig. 2. Clear-cell carcinoma characterized by a solid sheet of clear cells. H & E, × 170

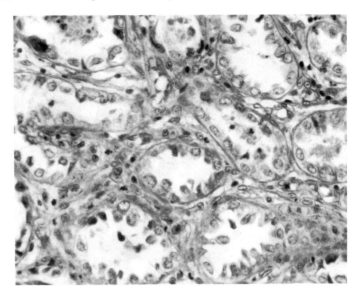

Fig. 3. Closely packed tubules lined by hobnail cells in a clear-cell carcinoma. H & E, × 400

a definite or probable history of DES exposure was elicited in 85% of the patients with vaginal tumors but only 66% of those with cervical tumors.

In the past these tumors had been designated mesonephric carcinoma [35, 36] because they were thought to be derived from mesonephric remnants, however, strong evidence now indicates that they are of müllerian origin. In the vagina and cervix the neoplasms are generally superficial and anterior [20, 22], whereas mesonephric remnants tend to lie deep in the lateral walls [25]. Secondly, although mesonephric remnants have been found in a few cases, these have been unrelated topographically to the vaginal and cervical neoplasms, whereas benign glandular structures of müllerian origin (adenosis and ectropion) are present either at the periphery of the tumor or admixed with it in almost all cases [20, 22]. Thirdly, the identical tumor occurs confined to the endometrium, a müllerian derivative [29, 44].

Almost one-quarter of the young women with clear-cell carcinomas of the vagina and cervix have either died or developed recurrent tumor, but this figure must still be regarded as tentative in view of the relatively short follow-up period in many of the cases [20, 22] (Table 3).

Factors related to survival include the size of the tumor, the depth of invasion, and the presence of lymph node metastasis [20, 22, 38]. Both radical surgery consisting of Wertheim hysterectomy and pelvic lymphadenectomy (including vaginectomy for patients with vaginal tumors) and radiation have been used effectively for patients with stage I and II vaginal tumors and stage I and IIA and IIB cervical lesions [20, 22].

Local resection has been advocated by some [51] for small superficial lesions; however, 17% of patients with stage I tumors of the cervix and vagina have pelvic lymph node metastasis and lymph node metastasis has occurred with tumors that have invaded only 1.5 mm [22]. Thus at the present time wide local excision cannot be recommended.

Clear-cell carcinoma appears to have a greater propensity for metastasis to the lungs and supraclavicular lymph nodes 35% frequency than squamous carcinoma of the vagina and cervix only 5%–10% [38].

Table 3. Survival after therapy [22][a]

Location stage	Number of patients	Number alive	Number with recurrence	Number dead	% Living
Vagina					
Stage I	65	54	7	4	83
Stage II	19	15	1	3	79
Stage III and IV	5	1	1	3	20
Subtotal	89	70	9	10	79
Cervix					
Stage I	23	22	0	1	95
Stage IIA	19	14	2	3	74
Stage IIB	14	8	0	6	57
Stage III and IV	9	3	2	4	33
Subtotal	65	47	4	14	72
Total patients: 154					

[a] A. L. HERBST et al.: Clear-cell adenocarcinoma of the vagina and cervix in girls: Analysis of 170 registry cases. Am. J. Obstet. Gynecol. *119*, 713—724 (1974).

Benign Alterations Associated with DES Exposure

Although the clear-cell carcinoma has received the widest attention, it is a relatively infrequent sequela of maternal DES treatment. In contrast almost all women exposed to DES will have one or more of the benign conditions, which include vaginal adenosis, cervical ectropion (erosion), and transverse vaginal and cervical ridges. An increasing number of terms has been used to describe these changes such as cervical pseudopolyp [19, 42], strawberry cervix [37], cervical cock's comblike lesion [37, 45], vaginal pericervical collar [19], vaginal hood [37, 45], and vaginal band [1], but these are all variants of the three basic lesions. Adenosis is characterized by benign glandular epithelium, either lining glands beneath the vaginal mucosa or replacing the surface epithelium [19, 28] (Figs. 4 and 5). Adenosis may appear clinically as a granular red patch or red stippling. It may be invisible if the glandular epithelium is replaced by immature squamous epithelium (squamous metaplasia), which often occurs. Since immature squamous epithelium is nonglycogenated, application of iodine results in nonstaining areas that stand out in sharp contrast to the typical glycogenated squamous epithelium of the vagina which appear dark brown with the absorbed iodine. Cervical ectropion is characterized by glandular epithelium on the exocervix (Fig. 6) and clinically has the same appearance as vaginal adenosis [19, 40]. Despite these apparent similarities between the two lesions, differences exist. The epithelium of vaginal adenosis may be mucinous (Fig. 5), resembling endocervical epithelium or be free of mucin and often ciliated (Fig. 7), resembling the epithelium of the endometrium or fallopian tube. In contrast, the epithelium of cervical ectropion resembles endocervical epithelium and usually lacks cilia [19]. The third benign lesion is the vaginal or cervical ridge (Fig. 8), which consists of a partial or complete band of fibroconnective tissue often covered by glandular epithelium. The ridge may be on the cervix or encircle the upper portion of the vagina, distorting the normal architecture and making it

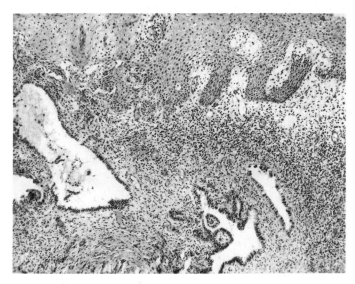

Fig. 4. Vaginal adenosis characterized by glands beneath the surface epithelium. A. L. HERBST et al.: Obstet. Gynecol. *40*, 287 (1972). H & E, × 90

extremely difficult to distinguish vagina from cervix [19, 40]. Variations in location and extent of the ridge and its relationship to the cervical ectropion account for the varied and imaginative terms used to describe these lesions. Thus if the ridge completely encircles the cervix, it has been called a pericervical collar [19]; if it is only partial and lies anterior to the cervix it has been called a hood [37, 45]. Occasionally the ridge is on the portio of the cervix and associated

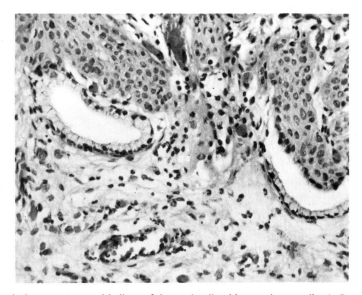

Fig. 5. Glands directly beneath the squamous epithelium of the vagina lined by mucinous cells. A. L. HERBST et al.: Obstet. Gynecol. *40*, 287 (1972) H & E, × 240

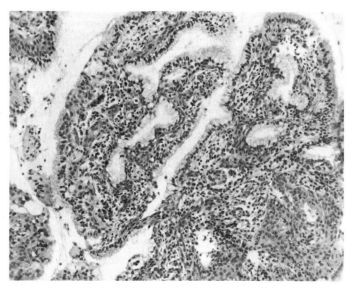

Fig. 6. Cervical ectropion characterized by papillary fronds lined by mucinous epithelium on the portio of the cervix. A. L. HERBST et al.: Obstet. Gynecol. *40*, 287 (1972). H & E, × 170

with an extensive cervical ectropion, giving the appearance of a large endocervical polyp protruding through the os. Careful probing will disclose that the true os is in the center of this "polyp" and consequently the term pseudopolyp has been proposed [19].

Although a definite transition between vaginal adenosis and clear-cell carcinoma has not been demonstrated, adenosis is closely associated with the tumor in 95% of the cases and probably

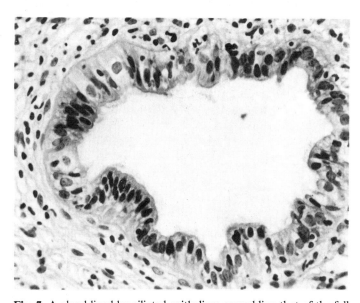

Fig. 7. A gland lined by ciliated epithelium resembling that of the fallopian tube and endometrium. A. L. HERBST et al.: Obstet. Gynecol. *20*, 287 (1972). H & E × 490

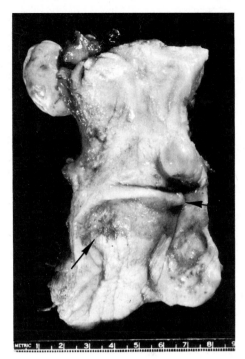

Fig. 8. Opened surgical specimen showing transverse cervical ridge (*arrow on right*) and extensive adenosis (*arrow on left*). A large nabothian cyst at right is present in the endocervical canal. A. L. HERBST et al.: New Engl. J. Med. *287*, 1259 (1972)

represents the source of the clear-cell adenocarcinoma of the vagina [20, 22] where glandular epithelium is normally not present. Likewise the cervical ectropion probably bears the same relationship to the cervical neoplasm [20, 22]. An almost constant, accompanying feature of adenosis is the presence of nests of immature to mature squamous epithelium replacing the

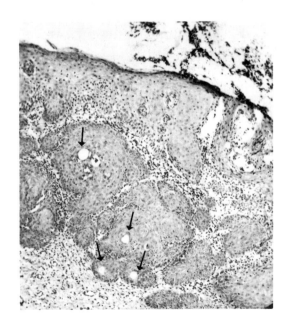

Fig. 9. Extensive squamous metaplasia replacing glands of vaginal adenosis. *Arrows* point to the remaining gland lumens. H & E, × 70

glands, which is referred to as squamous metaplasia [17, 19] (Fig. 9). When the process replaces all the glands in a microscopic section it may simulate a well-differentiated squamous carcinoma. However, the minimal atypia and the usual presence of both intracellular and extracellular mucin, demonstrated particularly well by mucin stains, indicate the non-neoplastic glandular nature of the nests. Squamous metaplasia appears to represent the healing phase of adenosis, ultimately replacing all the glandular epithelium and restoring a normal appearance to the vagina.

The finding of extensive areas of cervical ectropion and vaginal adenosis associated with squamous metaplasia has led some to conclude that one of the basic abnormalities of DES exposure is an aberrant location of the cervical transformation zone [46]. The latter is defined by colposcopists as an area characterized by squamous transformation (metaplasia) of columnar (glandular) epithelium. This zone is usually located on the exocervix in the vicinity of the external os and is the site of origin of most dysplasias and squamous cell carcinomas of the cervix. The presence of a large ectropion of the cervix or vaginal adenosis with consequent expansion of the transformation zone in DES-exposed women has led some colposcopists to speculate that there may be an increase in the incidence of squamous carcinoma in these individuals [6, 46]. At the present time this has not been realized, but continued careful surveillance of the at risk population will be necessary[1].

Since adenosis is believed to be the benign precursor of the clear-cell carcinoma, it is important to know the incidence of adenosis in the exposed population. HERBST et al. [21] have shown in a carefully matched prospective study that 35% of the group of exposed women had biopsy-proven adenosis compared to only 1% in the control group. Cervical ectropion was found in 85% of the exposed group and 38% of the controls. Transverse cervical and vaginal ridges were present in 22% of the exposed group and in none of the controls (Table 4).

As with the carcinoma, a relationship between these benign lesions and the dosage of DES could not be established. However, the frequency of these lesions was found to increase in an almost linear fashion, the earlier in pregnancy that DES treatment was initiated. Thus, if treatment was started prior to the 8th week of gestation, adenosis was found in 73% of patients and 100% had cervical ectropion. In contrast, if treatment began after the 17th week of gestation, vaginal adenosis was present in only 7% and cervical ectropion, in 70% (Table 5).

Table 4. Prevalence of benign abnormalities in DES-exposed and control populations[a]

Group	No.	Vaginal adenosis (%)	Cervical erosion (%)	Ridge (%)
Exposed	110	35	85	22
Control	82	1	38	0

[a] A. L. HERBST et al.: New Engl. J. Med. *292*, 334 (1975).

1 Since submission of this manuscript, a study of 1400 young women examined only because of a history of prenatal DES exposure revealed a 2.1% prevalence of dysplasia. The dysplastic process was almost always mild and tended to involve the cervix more frequently than the vagina. Moderate dysplasia occurred in only 3 of the 1400 patients and there were no examples of severe dysplasia or carcinoma in situ [38a].

Table 5. Frequency of benign abnormalities in relation to week of initiation of DES (133 patients)[a]

Wk.	No.	Vaginal adenosis (%)	Cervical erosion (%)	Ridge (%)
8	22	73	100	23
9—12	39	49	92	28
13—16	42	29	81	19
17	30	7	70	13

[a] A. L. HERBST et al.: New Engl. J. Med. *292*, 334 (1975).

Screening the Exposed Population

A large number of children and young women have been exposed to DES in utero and 15% of the patients in the Registry files were asymptomatic when their tumors were discovered. Moreover, in contrast to the survival of 75% for the entire group of patients, none of those that were asymtomatic at the time of diagnosis have died although the tumors recurred. The obvious question is whether or not all children and women with a history of exposure should undergo screening examinations. Since less than 10% of the patients with carcinoma have been under 12 years of age [22], it does not seem reasonable to subject exposed prepubertal children to multiple examinations, which require general anesthesia. Furthermore, only one-half of the patients in this age group in the Registry files had a history of DES exposure, so the others would not have been identified by screening examinations. Consequently it has been suggested that unless a prepubertal child has vaginal bleeding or discharge, pelvic examination can be deferred to the time of menarche or by the age of 14 years if the menarche has not occurred [22]. At this time all females with a history of DES exposure should be examined. The examination should include careful palpation and direct visualization supplemented with iodine staining. Colposcopy is a valuable adjunct for investigative purposes, but is not necessary for the detection of clear-cell carcinoma. Biopsy of all suspicious areas is mandatory as these tumors may be quite small and difficult to detect even with careful colposcopic examination. Cytology is a useful screening examination if the anterior, posterior, and lateral walls of the vagina are scraped [2, 31] but cannot be considered entirely reliable because of the relative frequency of false negative findings.

At the present time it does not appear necessary for male offspring of DES-treated mothers to be screened for malignant tumors as no increased incidence of neoplasms has been reported. The only alterations detected so far have been abnormalities of sperm including decreased counts, abnormal forms, and decreased mobility and small epididymal cysts [3].

References

1. Barber, H. R. K., Sommers, S. C.: Vaginal adenosis, dysplasia, and clear-cell adenocarcinoma after diethylstilbestrol treatment in pregnancy. Obstet. Gynecol. *43,* 645—652 (1974)
2. Bibbo, M., Ali, I., Al-Naqeeb, M., Baccarini, I., Climaco, L., Gill, W., Sonek, M., Weid, G. L.: Cytologic findings in female and male offspring of DES-treated mothers. Acta Cytol. *19,* 568—572 (1975)

3. Bibbo, M., Al-Naqeeb, M., Baccarini, I., Gill, W., Newton, M., Sleeper, K. M., Sonek, M., Weid, G. L.: Follow-up study of male and female offspring of DES-treated mothers. J. Rep. Med. *15*, 29—32 (1975)

4. Crosby, W. M., Hill, E. C.: Embryology of the müllerian duct system. Obstet. Gynecol. *20*, 507—515 (1962)

5. Dunn, T. B., Green, A. W.: Cysts of the epididymis, cancer of the cervix, granular cell myoblastoma, and other lesions after estrogen injection in newborn mice. J. Natl. Cancer Inst. *31*, 425—455 (1963)

6. Fetherston, W. C.: Squamous neoplasia of vagina related to DES syndrome. Am. J. Obstet. Gynecol. *122*, 176—180 (1975)

7. Fetherston, W. C., Meyers, A., Speckhard, M. E.: Adenocarcinoma of the vagina in young women. Wis. Med. J. *71*, 87—93 (1972)

8. Forsberg, J. G.: Effect of sex hormones on the development of the rat vagina. Acta Endocrinol. *33*, 520—531 (1960)

9. Forsberg, J. G.: Derivation and differentiation of the Vaginal Epithelium. Lund, Hakan Ohlssons Boktryker (1963)

10. Forsberg, J. G.: Estrogen, vaginal cancer and vaginal development. Am. J. Obstet. Gynecol. *113*, 83—87 (1972)

11. Forsberg, J. G.: Cervicovaginal epithelium: Its origin and development. Am. J. Obstet. Gynecol. *115*, 1025—1043 (1973a)

12. Forsberg, J. G.: Cervicovaginal epithelium: Its origin and development. Am. J. Obstet. Gynecol. *115*, 1025—1043 (1973b)

13. Greene, R. R., Burril, M. W., Ivy, A. C.: Experimental inter-sexuality. The paradoxical effects of estrogens on sexual development of the female rat. Anat. Rec. *74*, 429—438 (1939)

14. Greenwald, P., Barlow, J. J., Nasca, P. C., Burnett, W. S.: Vaginal cancer after maternal treatment with synthetic estrogens. New Engl. J. Med. *285*, 390—392 (1971)

15. Hameed, K.: Clear-cell "mesonephric" carcinoma of the uterine cervix. Obstet. Gynecol. *32*, 564—575 (1968)

16. Hart, W. R., Norris, H. J.: Mesonephric adenocarcinomas of the cervix. Cancer *29*, 106—113 (1972)

17. Hart, W. R., Townsend, D. E., Aldrich, J. O., Henderson, B. E., Roy, M., Benton, B.: Histopathologic spectrum of vaginal adenosis and related changes in stilbestrol-exposed females. Cancer *37*, 763—775 (1976)

18. Heinonen, O. P.: Diethylstilbestrol in pregnancy. Frequency of exposure and usage patterns. Cancer *31*, 573—577 (1973)

19. Herbst, A. L., Kurman, R. J., Scully, R. E.: Vaginal and cervical abnormalities after exposure to Stilbestrol in utero. Obstet. Gynecol. *40*, 287—298 (1972a)

20. Herbst, A. L., Kurman, R. J., Scully, R. E., Poskanzer, D. C.: Clear-cell adenocarcinoma of the genital tract in young females. Registry Report. New Engl. J. Med. *287*, 1259—1264 (1972b)

21. Herbst, A. L., Poskanzer, D. C., Robboy, S. J., Friedlander, L., Scully, R. E.: Prenatal exposure to stilbestrol. A prospective comparison of exposed female offspring with unexposed controls. New Engl. J. Med. *292*, 334—339 (1975)

22. Herbst, A. L., Robboy, S. J., Scully, R. E., Poskanzer, D. C.: Clear-cell adenocarcinoma of the vagina and cervix in girls: Analysis of 170 Registry cases. Am. J. Obstet. Gynecol. *119*, 713—724 (1974)

23. Herbst, A. L., Ulfelder, H., Poskanzer, D. C.: Adenocarcinoma of the vagina: Association of maternal stilbestrol therapy with tumor appearance in young women. New Engl. J. Med. *284*, 878—881 (1971)

24. Hill, E. C.: Clear-cell carcinoma of the cervix and vagina in young women. A report of six cases with association of maternal stilbestrol therapy and adenosis of the vagina. Am. J. Obstet. Gynecol. *116*, 470—481 (1973)

25. Huffman, J. W.: Mesonephric remnants in the cervix. Am. J. Obstet. Gynecol. *56*, 23–40 (1948)
26. Kantor, H. I., Weinstein, S. A., Kaye, H. L.: Clear-cell adenocarcinoma in young women. Obstet. Gynecol. *41*, 443–446 (1973)
27. Kurman, R. J., Craig, J. M.: Endometrioid and clear-cell carcinoma of the ovary. Cancer *29*, 1653–1664 (1972)
28. Kurman, R. J., Scully, R. E.: The incidence and histogenesis of vaginal adenosis. Hum. Pathol. *5*, 265–276 (1974)
29. Kurman, R. J., Scully, R. E.: Clear-cell carcinoma of the endometrium. An analysis of 21 cases. Cancer *37*, 872–882 (1976)
30. McLachlan, J. A., Newbold, R. R., Bullock, B.: Reproductive tract lesions in male mice exposed prenatally to diethylstilbestrol. Science *190*, 991–992 (1975)
31. Ng, A. B. P., Reagen, J. W., Hawliczek, S., Wentz, W. B.: Cellular detection of vaginal adenosis. Obstet. Gynecol. *46*, 323–328 (1975)
32. Noller, K. L., Decker, D. G., Lanier, A. P., Kurland, L. T.: Clear-cell adenocarcinoma of the cervix after maternal treatment with synthetic estrogens. Mayo Clin. Proc. *47*, 629–630 (1972)
33. Nordqvist, S. R. B., Fidler, W. J., Jr., Woodruff, J. M., Lewis, J. L., Jr.: Clear-cell adenocarcinoma of the cervix and vagina. A clinico-pathologic study of 21 cases with and without a history of maternal ingestion of estrogens. Cancer *37*, 858–871 (1976)
34. Norris, H. J., Robinowitz, M.: Ovarian adenocarcinoma of mesonephric type. Cancer *28*, 1074–1081 (1971)
35. Novak, E. R., Woodruff, J. D., Novak, E. R.: Probable mesonephric origin of certain female genital tumors. Am. J. Obstet. Gynecol. *68*, 1222–1239 (1954)
36. Novak, E. R., Woodruff, J. D.: Mesonephroma of the ovary. Thirty-five cases from the Ovarian Tumor Registry of the American Gynecological Society. Am. J. Obstet. Gynecol. *77*, 632–644 (1959)
37. Pomerance, W.: Post-stilbestrol secondary syndrome. Obstet. Gynecol. *42*, 12–18 (1973)
38. Robboy, S. J., Herbst, A. L., Scully, R. E.: Clear-cell adenocarcinoma of the vagina and cervix in young females: Analysis of 37 tumors that persisted or recurred after primary therapy. Cancer *34*, 606–614 (1974)
38a. Robboy, S. J., Keh, P. C., Nickerson, R. J., Helmanis, E. K., Prat, J., Szyfelbein, W. M., Taft, P. D., Barnes, A. B., Scully, R. E., Welch, W. R.: Squamous cell dysplasia and carcinoma in situ of the cervix and vagina after prenatal exposure to Diethylstilbestrol. Obstet. Gynecol. *51*, 528–535 (1978)
39. Roth, L. M., Hornback, N. B.: Clear-cell adenocarcinoma of the cervix in young women. Cancer *34*, 1761–1768 (1974)
40. Sandberg, E. C.: Benign cervical and vaginal changes associated with exposure to stilbestrol in utero. Am. J. Obstet. Gynecol. *125*, 777–788 (1976)
41. Scully, R. E., Barlow, J. F.: "Mesonephroma" of ovary. Tumor of müllerian nature related to the endometrioid carcinoma. Cancer *20*, 1405–1416 (1967)
42. Shane, J. M., Perlmutter, J. F.: Pseudopolyp of the uterine cervix. Am. J. Obstet. Gynecol. *115*, 273–274 (1973)
43. Silverberg, S. G., DeGiorgi, L. S.: Clear-cell carcinoma of the vagina: A clinical, pathologic, and electron microscopic study. Cancer *29*, 1680–1690 (1972)
44. Silverberg, S. G., DeGiorgi, L. S.: Clear-cell carcinoma of the endometrium. Clinical, pathologic and ultrastructural findings. Cancer *31*, 1127–1140 (1973)
45. Stafl, A., Mattingly, R. F., Foley, D. V., Fetherston, W. C.: Clinical diagnosis of vaginal adenosis. Obstet. Gynecol. *43*, 118–128 (1974a)
46. Stafl, A., Mattingly, R. F.: Vaginal adenosis: A precancerous lesion? Am. J. Obstet. Gynecol. *120*, 666–673 (1974b)
47. Taft, P. D., Robboy, S. J., Herbst, A. L, Scully, R. E.: Cytology of clear-cell adenocarcinoma of the genital tract in young females: Review of 95 cases from the Registry. Acta Cytol. *18*, 279–290 (1974)

48. Tsukada, Y., Hewett, W. J., Barlow, J. J., Pickren, J. W.: Clear-cell adenocarcinoma ("Mesoneph-roma") of the vagina: Three cases associated with maternal synthetic nonsteroid estrogen therapy. Cancer *29*, 1208–1214 (1972)
49. Ulfelder, H.: Stilbestrol, adenosis, and adenocarcinoma. Am. J. Obstet. Gynecol. *117*, 794–799 (1973)
50. Wells, L. J.: Embryology and anatomy of the vagina. Ann. N.Y. Acad. Sci. *83*, 80–88 (1959)
51. Wharton, J. T., Rutledge, F. N., Gallagher, H. S., Fletcher, G.: Treatment of clear-cell adenocarci-noma in young females. Obstet. Gynecol. *45*, 365–368 (1975)

Cancer and Other Lesions in Mice Receiving Estrogens

Thelma B. Dunn

Three papers in the Journal of the National Cancer Institute [4, 5, 7] provide a fairly complete list of references on this subject. The microscopic sections of material illustrated in my two papers are on file at the Registry of Experimental Cancers, National Cancer Institute (NCI) and can be examined there.

Diethylstilbestrol (DES)

The first paper describes experiments in which male and female mice from three groups were injected with diethylstilbestrol (DES) on the day of birth [5]. Lesions, which were probably related to the treatment, were found at autopsy in older mice. The female mice showed signs of continuous estrogen stimulation (Figs. 1—9).

The reason for injecting DES into newborn mice was that I was puzzled, and still am, by the curious distribution and types of tumors that appear when the polyoma virus, with which I was working, is injected into newborn mice. I thought that the newborn state might explain it. I and my assistant, an expert at handling newborns who attributed some of his success to wearing gloves rubbed in mouse litter before picking up the babies, began injecting them with almost anything that was handy. We injected many mice with DES and put them aside. When I returned from a Cancer Conference in Moscow, my assistant said that some of the female mice that had received DES had developed hard lumps in the lower abdomen. When these mice were autopsied at age 13 months, we found stones in the vaginas (Figs. 10 and 11). That same week a paper appeared from HOWARD BERN's laboratory in Berkeley, California, describing similar stones [11]. The explanation for these stones was that the urethra emptied into the vagina and the stones formed from the stagnant urine. Not all of the mice developed these stones. Many mice were maintained alive until they were more than 20 months of age. A variety of lesions were found at autopsy. Some males had "cysts" in the epididymis (Figs. 12—19). There were no other changes in the males and there was no evidence of an endocrine imbalance. McENTEE of Cornell University, Ithaca, New York, has found lesions described as "adenomyosis" in male dogs and bulls given estrogens (personal communication).

The findings in the female mice were more complex. A few had granular cell myoblastomas of the cervix or in the vaginal wall (Figs. 20 and 21). One of these was successfully transplanted and carried for several generations. This tumor is rare in men and in mice. SOBEL and MARQUET concluded that the human and the murine tumor are similar [10]. He tried to reproduce our work but reported to me that he could not get the newborn mice to survive the injections.

The most interesting finding was cancer of the cervix and vaginal wall (Figs. 22—29). These occurred most often in BALB/c mice. Two were successfully transplanted. Because of

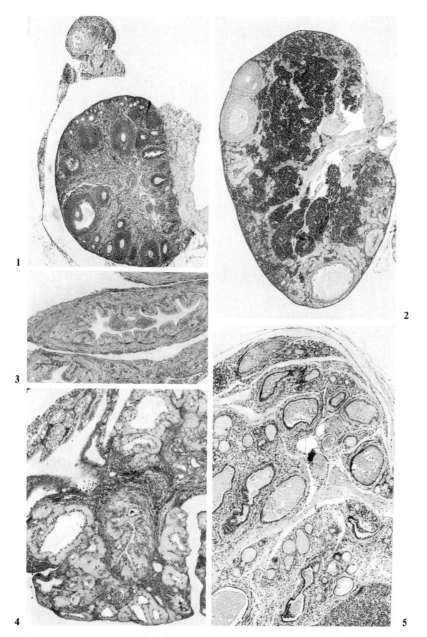

Fig. 1. Noninbred Swiss female mouse, age 3 months. *Ovary.* DES injected S.C. on day of birth. Note absence of corpora lutea. H & E, × 37

Fig. 2. BALB/c female mouse, age 14 months. *Ovary.* DES injected on day of birth. Note absence of corpora lutea, presence of cystic follicles, and abundant ceroid cells in medulla, heavily stained by the periodic acid-Schiff technique. × 37

Fig. 3. C3Hf female mouse, age 6 months. *Untreated. Uterine* tube showing secretory area. Cytoplasm of low columnar cells is clear, only faintly eosinophilic, and finely granular. Plump, oval nuclei are situated near center of cells. H & E, × 100

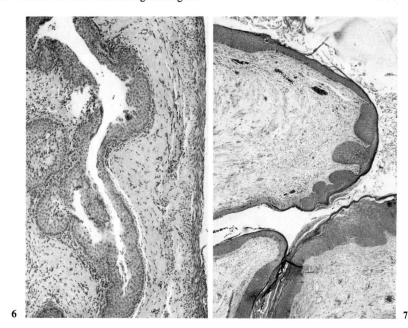

Fig. 6. BALB/c female mouse, age 14 months (same mouse as in Figure 2). *Uterus.* Note hyalinized endometrial stroma and epidermization of epithelium. H & E, × 95

Fig. 7. BALB/c female mouse, age 13 months. DES injected on day of birth. *Uterine cervix.* Note mucoid appearance of stroma and estrous type vaginal epithelium with slight proliferation at cervix. H & E, × 45

changes in the endometrium, the adrenals, the ovaries, and other organs, I considered these mice to be under a continuous estrogen stimulation. This prolonged stimulation was believed to explain the development of the cancers in older animals. BERN and his associates have also found cervical and vaginal cancers in very old mice injected with estrogens on the 5 successive days after birth [2]. Changes they termed "persistent vaginal cornification" were found consistently even in animals in which the ovaries and adrenals were removed or when altered vaginal epithelium was transferred to normal animals. Androgens given to newborn mice and rats produced similar lesions [8]. BERN's publications should be consulted for details of these experiments. A publication containing abstracts of papers presented at a seminar in Tokyo in 1972 entitled "Long-term Effects of Perinatal Hormone Administration" [12] is available in the Registry of Experimental Cancers at the NCI.

◀ **Fig. 4.** BALB/c female mouse, age 24 months. DES injected on day of birth. *Uterine tube* showing secretory area. Secretory cells are cuboidal, cytoplasm is eosinophilic, opaque, and dense, pyknotic nuclei lie at extreme tip. Nonsecretory portion shown in *upper left.* Compare with Figure 3. H & E, × 100

Fig. 5. BALB/c female mouse, age 19 months. DES injected on day of birth. *Mammary gland* tissue, secretory reaction. Ducts are dilated and contain eosinophilic secretion. H & E, × 70

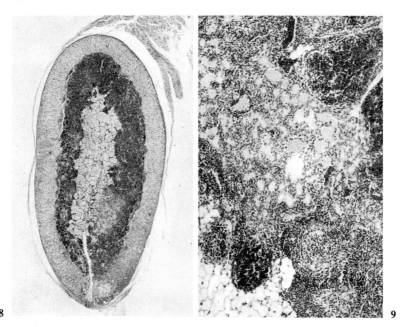

8   9

Fig. 8. BALB/c female mouse, age 19 months. DES injected on day of birth. *Adrenal gland.* Note wide zone of "brown degeneration", which stains deeply by the PAS technique. × 37

Fig. 9. BALB/c female mouse, age 24 months. DES injected on day of birth. *Thymus.* Note extreme atrophy and disappearance of lymphocytes. Multiple small cysts lined by flat cells with clear eosinophilic material are found within medulla. H & E, × 135

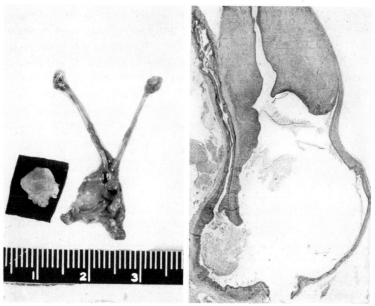

10   11

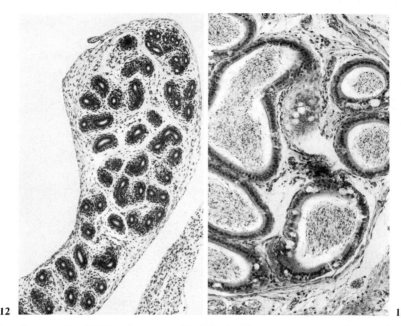

Fig. 12. *Untreated* newborn strain C3Hf male mouse. *Epididymis*. Note large amount of stromal connective tissue as compared to tubules. H & E, × 100

Fig. 13. Noninbred Swiss male mouse, age 2 months. DES injected on day of birth. *Epididymis*. Note that tubules are slightly dilated and many tubular lining cells are vacuolated. H & E, × 135

Interest in these experiments has increased recently because of the vaginal cancers found in young women whose mothers received DES during pregnancy. The cancers in the mice are epidermoid carcinomas, not adenocarcinomas. It is important to know whether or not the young women with these cancers have any evidence of hormonal imbalance and if they have an increased risk of other types of cancer in later life. Is the change in the vagina purely local? A recent report indicates that sons of mothers who received DES are often sterile and have epididymal cysts and other malformations of the genitalia [3].

More work needs to be done on this problem, but there may be many difficulties. When SNELL at the NCI attempted to inject rats with DES at different stages of pregnancy, many of the females aborted.

◄ **Fig. 10.** BALB/c female mouse, age 26 months. DES injected on day of birth. Dilated *vagina* has been opened, and stone is shown on *left*. On microscopic examination, an early cancer was seen at vaginal orifice. H & E, × 4

Fig. 11. C3Hf female mouse, age 24 months. DES injected on day of birth. Stone in vaginal cavity was decalcified before sectioning. *Urethra* on *left* empties into *vaginal cavity*. Precancerous lesion in vaginal mucosa just below urethral opening. Note downgrowths of epithelium in region of cervix. H & E, × 10

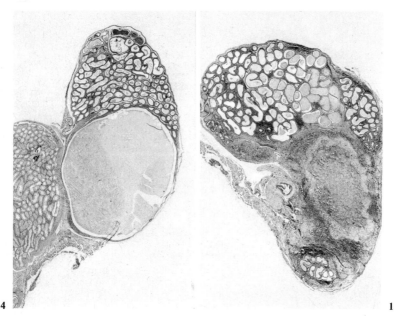

14   15

Fig. 14. BALB/c male mouse, age 26 months. DES injected on day of birth. *Epididymis* and *testis*. Note large cysts of epididymis. Testis is slightly atrophied, but many tubules appear normal and spermatocytes are found in tubules of epididymis. No interstitial cell increase in testis. H & E, × 10

Fig. 15. BALB/c male mouse, age 23 months. DES injected on day of birth. *Epididymis* and *testis*. Note that testis is replaced by fibrous tissue and tubules of epididymis are dilated. Testis on opposite side was not severely altered and epididymis contained a large spermatocele. H & E, × 15

Fig. 18. C3Hf male mouse, age 13 months. DES injected on day of birth. *Epididymis*. Note that tubules ▶ are dilated but do not appear cystic. Note increased interstitial tissue and some inflammatory reaction. H & E, × 43

Fig. 19. C3Hf male mouse, age 14 months. DES injected on day of birth. *Epididymis*. Note increase in interstitial tissue, moderate dilatation of tubules, and inflammatory reaction. H & E, × 100

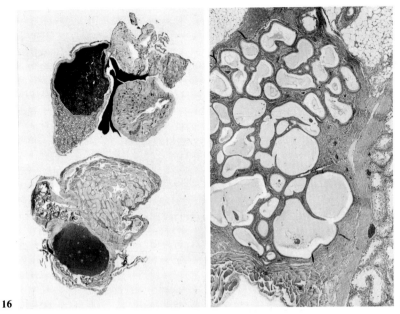

16
17

Fig. 16. BALB/c male mouse, age 26 months. DES injected on day of birth. *Epididymis* and *testis* from both sides are shown. Note bilateral cysts of epididymis, which contain heavily stained fluid. PAS, × 10

Fig. 17. BALB/c male mouse, age 13 months. DES injected on day of birth. *Epididymis* and *testis*. Note multiple small cysts of epididymis and fairly normal testicular tubules on *right*. H & E, × 37

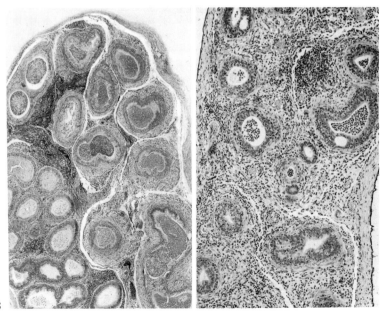

18
19

182 Thelma B. Dunn

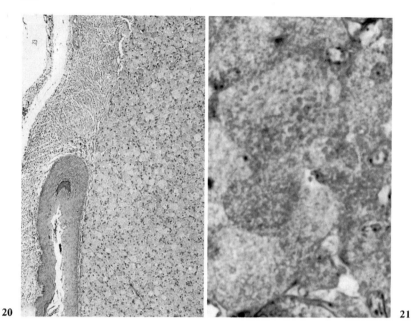

20   21

Fig. 20. BALB/c female mouse, age 26 months. DES injected on day of birth. Margin of uterine *cervix* with granular cell myoblastoma just beneath epithelial surface. H & E, × 70

Fig. 21. Higher magnification of granular cell myoblastoma. Note granulation and abundant cytoplasm of tumor cells. Cell margins are obscured by heavily stained granules that vary in quantity and size in different cells. PAS, × 880

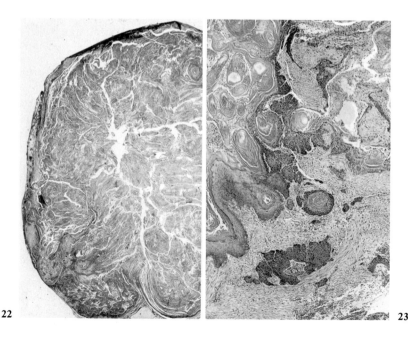

22   23

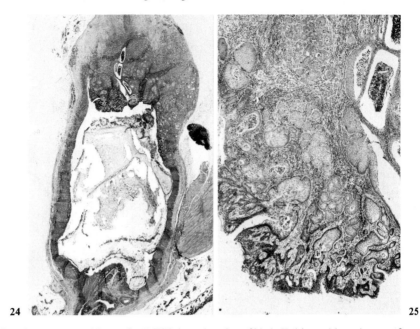

Fig. 24. BALB/c female mouse, age 21 months. DES injected on day of birth. Epidermoid carcinoma of *cervix* and decalcified stone in vagina. H & E, × 10

Fig. 25. Higher magnification of *cervical* cancer shown in Figure 24. Note atrophy of vaginal epithelium above cancerous downgrowth of epidermoid tissue. H & E, × 50

◄ **Fig. 22.** BALB/c female mouse, age 20 months. DES injected on day of birth. Cross section of *vagina,* filled with necrotic squamous material formed by *epidermoid cancer.* Site of origin within cavity could not be determined. No stone found. Cancer successfully transplanted. H & E, × 6

Fig. 23. Higher magnification of cancer of *vaginal wall* shown in Figure 22. Note infiltration of muscle wall. H & E, × 50

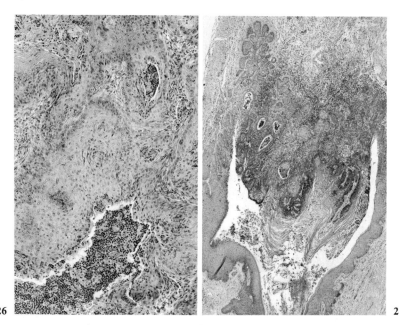

26   27

Fig. 26. BALB/c female mouse, age $2\frac{1}{3}$ months. Transplanted with epidermoid carcinoma of *vagina* when 1 month old. Note collections of granulocytes within epidermoid epithelial spaces. H & E, × 150

Fig. 27. C3Hf female mouse, age 26 months. DES injected on day of birth. Epidermoid carcinoma of the *cervix*. Note infiltration of submucosal tissue, estrous state of vaginal epithelium, and absence of stone formation. H & E, × 37

Enovid

Enovid (mestranol and norethynodrel) injected into mice appeared to have an effect similar to DES, but the changes were less severe and less constant than those that occurred in mice that received DES [4]. Enovid was also given in a liquid diet to assure continuous ingestion of the drug. This experiment followed a meeting at the NCI at which the first trials of Enovid in women were described by PINCUS. When I asked about the effects of this drug on animals, I was told that it would not act as a contraceptive in animals. At the same meeting, changes were reported in the livers of rats given very high doses of the drug.
The BALB/c mice in our laboratory were given a dose of Enovid that I calculated would sterilize them. Although the Enovid was mixed with a powdered feed, it proved to be extremely difficult to maintain mice by this method. Because the mice continued to breed, the dose was doubled. They still continued to breed and the dose was doubled again, but they were still not sterile. Other investigators whom I consulted, who had given Enovid to mice in powdered food, had had similar experiences.
Enovid did effectively induce sterility, however, when given in a liquid diet. Advantages to the liquid diet are many. It is easy to measure the amount of liquid consumed and the desired dosage of a drug is easily altered. GREENSTEIN (see reference in [4]) had tried before to

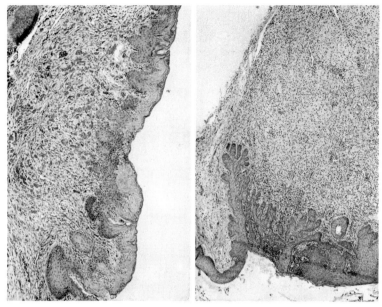

28   29

Fig. 28. C3Hf female mouse, age 26 months. DES injected on day of birth. Epidermoid carcinoma in wall of *vagina* near orifice. Note infiltration by small nests of epidermal cells and atrophy of mucosa at site of origin. Cancer was also found in the *cervix* of this mouse. H & E, × 70

Fig. 29. C3Hf female mouse, age 24 months. DES injected on day of birth. Lesion at *cervix* considered *precancerous*. Note atrophic vaginal epithelium over area of downgrowth of epithelial cells. A stone was found in vagina. H & E, × 100

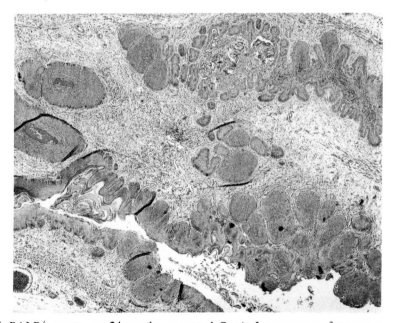

Fig. 30. Virgin female BALB/c mouse, age 24 months, *untreated. Cervix.* Large masses of squamous epithelial cells shown *below* result from infolding of surface epithelium and may simulate proliferation. Dyskeratotic lesion above. *Uterus* is toward *left.* H & E, × 125

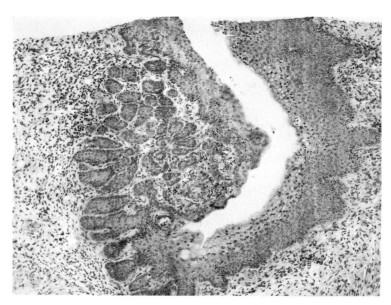

Fig. 31. Virgin female BALB/c mouse, age 18.5 months. Enovid injected S.C. on day of birth. Epithelial extensions in *cervix* which are little, if any, more extreme than in untreated mice. Uterus is toward *left*. H & E, × 125

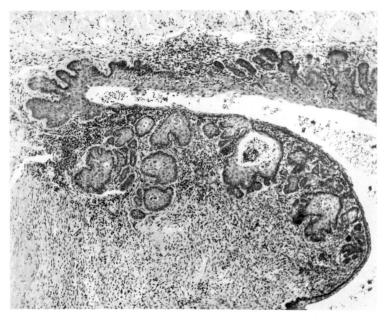

Fig. 32. Virgin female BALB/c mouse, 28 months old. Enovid injected on day of birth. Early *cervical cancer*. Cysts lined by well-differentiated stratified squamous epithelium containing desquamated cells and chromatin debris. Cysts extend into vaginal stroma, which also shows granulocytic infiltration. H & E, × 125

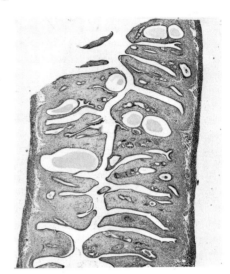

Fig. 33. BALB/c mouse fed Metrecal-Enovid from 95–721 days of age. *Uterus.* Note characteristic hyalinization of endometrial stroma, reduction in number of glands, and cystic dilatation. H & E, × 25

produce a synthetic diet for mice and had kept them alive for several months. We kept one group of mice alive for 8 months on fresh grade A milk and killed them when they developed a severe anemia. Metrecal, a dietary supplement manufactured by Mead Johnson Nutritionals, bought on the open market, was chosen for the vehicle because it was the most convenient. We found that with Metrecal the teeth did not grow to an excessive length and the feces formed normally. The mice did not weigh as much as controls on food pellets, but they appeared healthy. On liquid diet the food must be changed daily and the mice require more supervision than mice consuming pellets; this is perhaps also a positive feature because experiments involve many more mice than can be properly examined by the limited number of trained pathologists now available. Another advantage is that a highly toxic substance can be more safely handled in a liquid food. MUNOZ began an experiment in Lyon using Metrecal, Enovid,

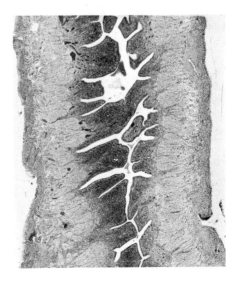

Fig. 34. BALB/c mouse, born to mother receiving Metrecal alone. This mouse was fed Metrecal until it was killed at age 598 days. Note size of uterus compared to mouse fed Enovid. Endometrium and muscular coats are normal. H & E, × 25

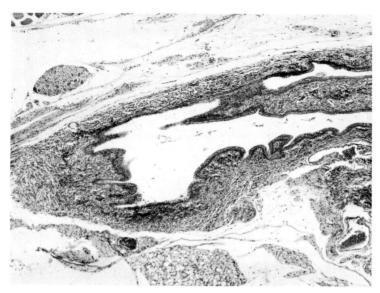

Fig. 35. Control BALB/c mouse fed Metrecal alone from birth to 550 days. *Cervix* shows no keratinization and no epithelial extensions. *Uterus* lies on the *left*. H & E, × 65

and a herpesvirus to try to induce cervical cancer. After ∼ 1 year, mice receiving Metrecal alone suddenly began to die, whereas those receiving Enovid were outliving the controls. At autopsy, the mice receiving Metrecal had auricular thrombi in the hearts which had caused death. A paper from the laboratory of WILLIAMS [1] described similar thrombi in mice on a

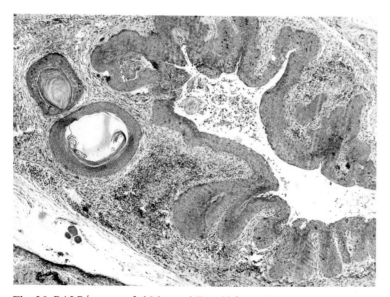

Fig. 36. BALB/c mouse fed Metrecal-Enovid from 105–518 days. Note thickening of *cervical* and *vaginal* epithelium and cystic extensions into cervical stroma. *Uterus* lies on the *left*. H & E, × 65

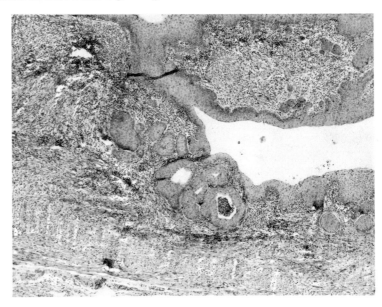

Fig. 37. BALB/c mouse fed Enovid from 105—518 days. *Cervix.* Note cystic extensions into stroma. H & E, × 65

high-fat, low-protein diet. Pregnant mice were more affected. This explained why the mice receiving Enovid survived longer. Obviously the Metrecal that MUNOZ was using was not the same that I had used. This fiasco shows the need for a standardized liquid food designed for mice.

The mice receiving the Enovid in Metrecal were sterile and showed signs of continuous estrogen stimulation. When older, they developed small cancers of the uterine cervix that did not extend outside the uterus or vagina nor did they metastasize (Figs. 30—40). Consequently these cancers were not recognized during gross inspection at autopsy and transplantations were not attempted. No cancers were found in any other organs except those expected in this strain. No cervical cancers were found in the controls on Metrecal alone. Much more work should be done and a properly balanced liquid food would be useful. We must answer several questions. Would there be a difference in response if the Enovid feeding were started at an early age in comparison with a later age? Could the Enovid be given for a limited period and cause no trouble later on? Would the cervical cancers be transplantable if an attempt were made?

The paper by HESTON et al. [7] describes experiments in which Enovid was incorporated into food pellets. It was given at three dose levels to five strains of mice. Only the highest dose prevented pregnancy and the response varied in the different strains. Whereas cervical cancer was found almost exclusively in BALB/c mice, pituitary tumors were found only in C57BL mice. No increase in mammary or ovarian tumors was found. The number of hepatomas in C3H/fB mice was actually less in Enovid-fed mice than in controls. This difference may be explained by the smaller size of the Enovid-treated mice, because good nutrition seems to promote the development of hepatomas in mice.

My only disagreements with HESTON's work are that the microscopic sections were not examined by a pathologist. Also his statement that spontaneous cervical cancer is so frequent

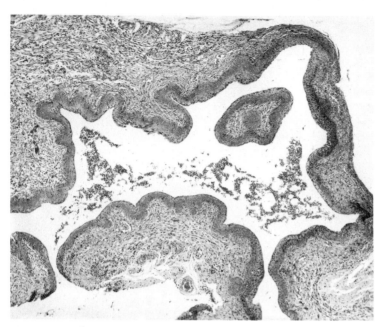

Fig. 38. BALB/c mouse fed Metrecal alone from 105—645 days. *Cervix* and *vagina* are normal. H & E, × 65

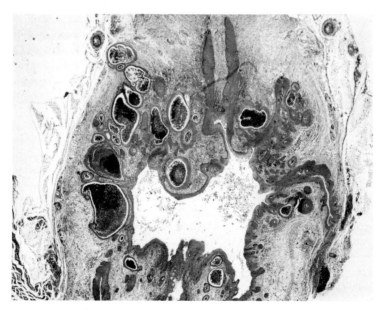

Fig. 39. BALB/c mouse fed Metrecal-Enovid 105—731 days. *Uterine cervix* and *vagina* containing infiltrating cervical carcinoma. Note cystic extensions into cervical stroma. Cysts at *left* extend through cervical stroma and reach almost to ureter. Uterus lies *above*. H & E, × 20

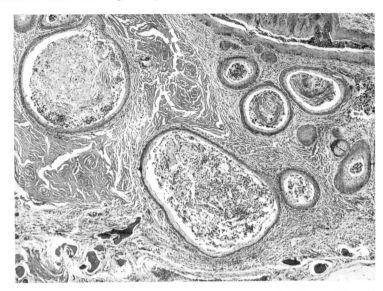

Fig. 40. BALB/c mouse, born to mother fed Metrecal-Enovid. This mouse was fed Metrecal-Enovid until it was killed at age 666 days. Note cysts lined with squamous epithelium, often containing squamous cells and chromatin debris. Unusual feature is amorphous, hyaline, mucoid substance in stroma of cervix. H & E, × 65

in BALB/c mice as to be of little use in studies of cervical cancer is contrary to my experience and that of others. Cervical cancer is very rare in mice, but changes occur in the cervix of old mice that can be mistaken for cancer. HESTON observed, as I had, that the cancers were of microscopic size, did not metastasize, and were not very invasive. A statement in HESTON's paper reads as follows: "Results from experimental animals should be applied to man with care, especially in this area where the use of antifertility drugs is so greatly needed in controlling probably the world's greatest problem — overpopulation". All would probably agree with this statement, but the danger of overpopulation should not influence the conduct of experiments with antifertility drugs.

Conclusions

Estrogens have different effects on rodents of different species. Female mice of some strains develop granular cell myoblastomas and cancers of the cervix and vagina. Under certain conditions they develop mammary cancers, but this is so complicated that I will not go into it here but refer the reader to the book "Neoplastic Development" by FOULDS [6], which gives an excellent analysis of the various factors. Male mice develop interstitial cell tumors of the testes. Female mice of some strains develop pituitary tumors. Estrogens also act as cocarcinogens, as witnessed by MURPHY's finding that the induction of cervical cancer by 3-methylcholanthrene was more rapid if estrogen was administered [9]. Rats develop mammary tumors. Male hamsters have kidney tumors. Female guinea pigs develop hormone-dependent tumors that resemble human fibromyomas in the wall of the uterus and within the abdominal cavity which regress when estrogen is discontinued. Female rabbits develop mammary and uterine tumors.

The great variation among rodents shows how unpredictable the carcinogenic effects of estrogen may be and how dubious it would be to apply these findings directly to human beings. But it also shows that whenever they are adequately tested, estrogens have proved to be carcinogens. Estrogens as potential carcinogens warrant much more attention than they have received so far. When we consider the current degree of exposure of the human population, many more carefully supervised animal experiments involving many more species under varying conditions should be performed.

All photographs were previously published in the Journal of the National Cancer Institute.

References

1. Ball, C. R., Clower, B. R., Williams, W. L.: Dietary induced atrial thrombosis in mice. Arch. Pathol. *80,* 391–396 (1965)
2. Bern, H. A., Jones, L. A., Mills, K. T., Kohrman, A., Mori, T.: Use of the neonatal mouse in studying long-term effects of early exposure to hormones and other agents. J. Toxicol. Environ. Health, Suppl. *1,* 103–116 (1976)
3. Bibbo, M., Gill, W. B., Azizi, F., Blough, R., Fang, V. S., Rosenfield, R. L., Schumacher, G. F. B., Sleeper, K., Sonek, M. G., Wied, G. L.: Follow-up study of male and female offspring of DES-exposed mothers. Obstet. Gynecol. *49,* 1–8 (1977)
4. Dunn, T. B.: Cancer of the uterine cervix in mice fed a liquid diet containing an antifertility drug. J. Natl. Cancer Inst. *43,* 671–692 (1969)
5. Dunn, T. B., Green, A. W.: Cysts of the epididymis, cancer of the cervix, granular cell myoblastoma and other lesions after estrogen injection in newborn mice. J. Natl. Cancer Inst. *31,* 425–455 (1963)
6. Foulds, L.: Neoplastic Development. London and New York: Academic Press, Vol. 2, 1975
7. Heston, W. E., Vlahakis, G., Desmukes, B.: Effects of the antifertility drug, Enovid, in five strains of mice, with particular regard to carcinogenesis. J. Natl. Cancer Inst. *51,* 209–224 (1973)
8. Kimura, T., Nandi, S.: Nature of induced persistent vaginal cornification in mice. IV. Changes in the vaginal epithelium of old mice treated neonatally with estradiol or testosterone. J. Natl. Cancer Inst. *39,* 75–93 (1967)
9. Murphy, E. D.: Carcinogenesis of the uterine cervix in mice. Effect of diethylstilbesterol after limited application of 3-methylcholanthrene. J. Natl. Cancer Inst. *27,* 611–653 (1961)
10. Sobel, H. J., Marquet, E.: Granular cells and granular cell lesions. In: Pathology Annual. Sommers, S. C. (Ed.). New York: Appleton-Century-Crofts, 1974, p. 43
11. Takasugi, N., Bern, H. A.: Crystals and concretions in the vaginae of persistent-estrous mice. Proc. Soc. Biol. Med. *109,* 622–624 (1962)
12. Takewaki, K., Bern, H. A.: Seminar on long-term effects of perinatal hormone administration. Tokyo, The International House of Japan (1972)

Subject Index

Recent Results in Cancer Research

Sponsored by the Swiss League against Cancer. Editor in Chief: P. Rentchnick, Genève